A Better Normal

Your Guide to Rediscovering Intimacy After Cancer

Tess Devèze

Jessa & Emmy, this one's on you.

CONTENTS

Part 3: Let's get sexy

Where to from here?

ACKNOWLEDGEMENTS

For anyone and everyone out there affected by cancer, this book is for you. There can be so much to consider, to have to endure, to have to keep track of, that many parts of life take a back seat. Thank you for caring about your intimacy and connections during such a time, be it connections with yourself or with others. I hope you're supported and I truly hope there is something in this book for you.

I'm forever grateful to my clients and the thousands I support online who so openly and vulnerably share their struggles, and also their triumphs with me. This book would not exist without you. I'm inspired and amazed by you all, daily.

Thank you, to my partners and carers Rog & Robi, my family and my global network of friends. There were some very dark places during treatments and you all got me through. To my booby buddies (my breast care nurses) Claire & Monique, you're my angels. Ricky Dick my oncologist - you're simply the best (Tina Turner style!) and to my RADelaidies.

Lastly, to acknowledge the incredible ethics, values and approaches to sexuality and communication from Roger Butler at Curious Creatures (and their generosity with sharing their content with me), the occupational therapy & sexuality community (yeah OT-siggers!) and the revolutionary perspectives and therapeutic trainings I received from Deej & Uma, at the Institute of Somatic Sexology (ISS).

WHY I WROTE THIS BOOK

Hello! It's so wonderful to meet you. I'm Tess.

I thought before we get into the more 'intimate' details, I'd introduce myself and let you know what this book is about.

I was diagnosed with stage-three breast cancer in 2018, at the age of 36. At the time of my diagnosis, I'd been working in the sexuality sector for years. Over the years since my cancer diagnosis and endless treatments, only twice did a healthcare professional voluntarily bring up the topic of sexuality and only one booklet was recommended to me (which I had to go and find myself). The lack of information and support on this topic, both during and after treatments, was painfully noticeable.

Why aren't more resources available? Why are we so afraid to talk about this essential aspect of our lives?

First and foremost, I'm an occupational therapist (OT). What's an OT, I hear you ask? We are functional therapists who help our clients with independence and participation in any kind of meaningful life activity ('occupation'). OTs help you accomplish the day-to-day activities that are important to you, as best you can. This may include self-care tasks (shower, dressing, toileting), work related (vocational) tasks, social or community activities…and may also include sex!

My clinical experience is mostly in sexuality - during and

after cancer treatments, brain-injury, neurological conditions, and those living with disability. Before moving solely to sexuality for people with cancer, disability and chronic illness, most of my work was in private and public hospitals across Australia, working in neurological rehabilitation. I love neuroscience, and most of the themes in this book are based on neurological concepts. I'm smiling as I type this, because I imagine you might be confused: "I want to learn about sex & intimacy, not neuroscience!" But hear me out! I promise, if you stick with me, you'll learn a *lot*.

Other than having cancer and being a sexuality OT, I also work with sexuality and self-development pioneers Curious Creatures, based in Melbourne Australia. I've facilitated well over 100 workshops online and face to face for nearing a decade, teaching consent, better intimacy and communication skills. I've seen thousands of people's lives change through a deeper understanding of sexual intimacy.

Lastly, I've also studied sexological bodywork at the Institute of Somatic Sexology. This training has given me a deeper understanding of how libido, pleasure, arousal and orgasmicity (cool word huh?) work on a physiological, neurological, and psychological level. These learnings form an essential part of this book.

Over the years, I've observed the way cancer affected my relationships with the people around me. Throughout all of my treatments (chemo, radio, surgeries, endocrine/hormone treatments), my sexuality and intimacy has suffered. And it suffered differently with each treatment.

Even with all my training, I've struggled. If you're struggling too, you're not alone. We all struggle (even if it doesn't get spoken about).

Over the past few years, I've really put my skills and training to the test, and sexually rehabilitated myself after each of my treatments. This book details not only my insights as someone fighting cancer, but also a decade of training, clinical expertise and experience.

But it's not just about me. The contents of this book are also guided by you. I have a Facebook group with thousands of people - all cancers, all genders - from over 43 countries, who share and support each other on this topic. My one-on-one clients have also been a huge source of learning, generously sharing their experiences.

I've written this book to help cancer patients and their loved ones maintain and grow connection, intimacy and sexuality. For those fighting or living with cancer, things like connection, love, support, and intimacy can be incredibly important. Humans are connective, social creatures; our relationships influence our wellbeing, happiness and resilience. Unfortunately, treatments and their side effects often make maintaining these connections much more complicated. If you've received a cancer diagnosis, or are the loved one of someone who has, this book shares ways to increase connection and intimacy with the important people in your life. Aside from making life more enjoyable, I see them as allies to our coping and to the recovery process.

This book is for all human beings, regardless of gender, lifestyle, orientation, ability, ethnicity, age, or relationship dynamic. Although every person with cancer is unique, we have one thing in common: no matter who we are or what we are going through, we're all worthy of love and connection.

This book is split into three main parts:

- **Part 1** clarifies the language I use, and some core information regarding intimacy, communication and libido.

- **Part 2** covers strategies to connect with those around you around various treatments and side-effects, how to recover pleasure and desire, and specific examples and activities for connecting with family, friends, carers and partners.

- **Part 3** addresses the more intimate topics such as how to communicate about sexuality, navigate positioning, loss of pleasure, vaginal pain and other tips and tricks regarding intimacy so you can reconnect.

To finish, I've listed some resources for further support, as you know, info on this topic is hard to find.

Many cancer patients tell me that when the more intensive treatments are over, they feel unsupported around getting back into everyday life. It's as if they've been released back into the wild, wide-eyed and alone, to figure out how to survive in what's often referred to as the 'new normal'. I personally can't stand those words! To me, 'new normal' feels as if we're being told we need to accept that life will never be the same. We feel as though we need to suck it up and get on with it. But I don't accept that. The 'new normal' can feel rotten at times, and it doesn't have to be that way. I know things can be better! And through the strategies and supports in this book, 'the new normal' can be better for you too.

This isn't one-size-fits-all advice. All bodies are unique, every relationship is different, and everyone experiences relationships, connection, pleasure and desire in their own way. You're the expert on you! Just as cancer is different for everyone, so are the connections we have with ourselves and those around us. So please don't feel obligated to read this start to finish...choose the sections which feel applicable to you.

The most important things you can learn from this book are that you're not alone and you're not broken. There's nothing wrong with you if you're struggling. It's normal to find this situation tough. Look at what cancer treatments do to us!

The stress, the anxiety, the chemicals, the pain, the fatigue, the toxins…if your body didn't have side-effects and you didn't experience changes in your body and intimacy, *that* would be the strange thing.

Now, let's get started on making your 'new normal', a 'better normal'.

PART 1: THE NUTS AND BOLTS

Tess Devèze

When you reach the end of Part 1, you should have a simple understanding of the language and key terms used in this book regarding sexuality, along with the foundational themes around libido and communication.

What I cover in this section

- What the words 'sexuality' and 'sex' actually mean.
- The difference between libido and arousal.
- What intimacy and connection are, and the vital role they play in our lives.
- How the 'spontaneity' of sex can be missed, however is not the end of your intimacy.
- Understanding what libido is and how it works in our body, so we can then work on its recovery.
- Why communication is difficult, but so important with some practical tools.
- Acknowledgement and support for the LGBTQIA+ community.

1. KEY TERMS EXPLAINED

Sexuality vs sex

The word 'sexuality' is an umbrella term which yes includes the functional activity of sex, but also includes relationships, connections, affection, dating, pleasure and our overall well-being. Sexuality can be greatly affected due to cancer, but it doesn't necessarily have to stop altogether. As a sexuality educator and clinician, I know how important sexuality, connection and intimacy is to our quality of life, our resilience and coping. What could be more important!

'Sex' in this book refers to the act, or the activity you engage in with yourself and/others, and is one of the most diverse and most adaptable functional activities I can think of. Yet today, it's still one of the most under-addressed topics in clinical settings. This is something I aim to change.

I also want us all to be on the same page in how we see 'sex' itself which is more than just orgasms and genital play, it's so much more. During cancer treatments and other life-altering events, you might need to temporarily let go of traditional forms of touch/sex. We can become excited, aroused, release pleasure hormones in our body from so many different ways. There are erogenous zones all over our bodies such as our inner thighs, breasts, nipples, under the armpits, the neck, earlobes, feet and many more depending on your body.

Orgasms, engorgement, ejaculation, becoming 'hard' or 'wet', these don't need to be your goal, but can also be experienced in more than one way. Pleasure, enjoyment, arousal, excitation and connection, that is where the fun can also be. Pleasure is pleasurable and our whole body can be pleasured!

Desire vs arousal

Desire (the wanting) I use interchangeably with libido. Desire/libido are the experience of *wanting* sex and pleasure. Desire has many words that can be used, such as lust, sex-drive, and essentially all refer to that *want* we have.

Arousal is the way our body responds when it's in pleasure, the changes in our body that show us we are in fact, enjoying and excited. Things like increased sensitivity, maybe we become wet, maybe we become hard, our heart rate increases, we breathe heavier and more.

Treatments can affect our arousal as well as our libido, which I dive into in this book, but knowing the difference between these can be very helpful.

The magical word, intimacy

Disconnection is a common side-effect of cancer treatments for so many. You're not alone in this and here I introduce you to the magical word 'intimacy'. Imagine that you having sex or being intimate again with yourself, a date or a partner/s, is the goal or the prize. That prize is on the other side of a river, and to get to it, you need to build a bridge. How can you do that? Through intimacy, through touch and the other magical word *affection*.

I've heard many times from clients and people in my support group "we don't even touch each other anymore". Not only has sex gone, but so has the *intimacy*, and are we really going to want sex without that connection?

Intimacy and affection are small giants. Tiny little things that can mean the world, and build that bridge of connection. Things like hand-holding, a good-night kiss, a good morning hug, your arm around your partner in the kitchen, cuddling on the couch, touch for the sake of touch (not as a way to 'get somewhere'), massage swaps, maybe a cheeky butt-squeeze and grin, and the big one, WORDS OF LOVE.

When you want some touch or love? Here's a few ways to ask, without that pressure of it needing to lead to sex:

How to say it out loud.

- "Hey, I'd like to be closer to you, how about a cuddle?"
- "Can we snuggle together on the couch while watching this film?"
- "You up for some hand-holding while we walk to the shop?"
- "I'm loving you right now, thought I'd share."

- "You up for some underwear-on cuddling while we fall asleep? I miss connecting with you."

- "I'd love some touch/to touch your body, would you like a massage?"

- "I'm not wanting this to lead to sex, but some kisses and cuddles would be lovely if you're feeling like some connection?"

- "I'm checking you out right now, just wanted to share."

- "I'm running a bath to relax and wind-down from the day, would you like to join me for some down-time?"

Small giant steps towards that prize.

2. CONNECTION

When people hear the word 'connection', some assume it means something to do with sex. Well, that is not necessarily always the case as there are so many different types of meaningful connection in our lives, which I'll discuss here.

Connection could be the sharing of intimacy through affection with another, or with yourself. It can make you warm, bring you closer to someone, provide feelings of value and being loved. A hug from a friend, a hand-hold from a family member, even a simple smile from a stranger. Connection, belonging, it all can have a positive impact on us.

Have you heard of the hormone oxytocin? It's referred to as the 'cuddle hormone'. Not only is this hormone released in the body during arousal, but softer, slower forms of touch, such as hand holding or cuddles (just to name a few) can also produce this pleasure hormone. This proves that you can still feel connected, even from the simplest forms of touch such as a hug or soft kiss on the cheek.

There will be relationships and connections in your life that become distant after a diagnosis and there are many reasons for this. Some relationships will struggle, some will fail, some simply might not understand how unwell you are and others might leave or pull away. I lost people during my treatments; people very close to me. I was not coping at all; I was struggling while trying to survive and put walls around me. It's sad, but not an uncommon story. Remember, one of the most difficult things you can experience during treatment is the challenge of putting yourself first. You're fighting for your life, you must. It's how you will manage to face each day. It's how you will survive. Know that other relationships can get stronger, deeper, more loving and connected, and you may even end up with stronger supports and connections around you than before. For some, it can be described as a reshuffle of love. I'm here to help you with the reshuffle and with making deeper connections.

Why connecting is essential

I want to share a 'light bulb' moment I had during chemotherapy, one that helped me change a lot about the way I connected to those around me.

I was 4 months into chemotherapy and had just switched to having chemo weekly. It was a sweltering 38-degree Australian summer night and I walked out of a poetry reading with a friend, to go home. While walking, he hooked his arm through mine, as a sign of affection and connection. When his arm linked through mine, I noticed that I jumped at the touch. Noticing my reaction and how much I had been startled at the contact, it dawned on me. How long had it been since I had been touched in a way that was not medical, hurried and detached? Three weeks? Maybe four? I was so used to the non-intimate hands of nurses, oncologists, surgeons etc. who were not aggressive, but let's say, purposefully unaffectionate in their touch. It was a shock to receive this wonderful soft, intimate connection of an arm slipping through mine. I realised I had become an object of analysis and procedure, and was no longer one of affection. It was shocking to me and it also saddened me.

That was the moment I realised I was losing connection, that was the moment I saw I was becoming detached and I needed to be more vocal. The people around me were being respectful and careful not to touch me, due to how unwell I was. I loved everyone's respectful approach and care towards me as I was very, very sick. I'm grateful for their care, but I realised they also needed guidance from me, to know what was okay and when.

Realising the only touch I had been receiving was medical, which I would switch off to and detach myself from, was one of those 'ahaaa' moments. I had realised how disconnected I had become to my body and that I needed to make the first move and communicate. So, I beg you, educate those around you. Tell your friends they can hold your hand, your family members can put their arm around you, a partner or lover can snuggle with you on the couch. Be their guide for your connection. There are some examples on how to do that further on in this section.

Our desires for physical intimacy change when we are stressed and unwell, that is a part of being human. However, it's important to mention here that treatments and the endless medications we take around it, can also affect our mind. 'Cancer-brain' also known as 'brain-fog' is actual cognitive dysfunction. It was and is, one of the most challenging side effects for me. Being unable to think, remember, concentrate, getting lost in my apartment building, losing my keys, forgetting the names of loved ones, it was and is scary. So, how do we give an invisible symptom, visibility? We speak of it, we give it voice, we give others' knowledge and understanding. It was difficult, however was helpful for the people around me.

When I described to my friends how upsetting it was, that I couldn't remember what we were talking about minute to minute, or how angry I was that I couldn't focus on more than one conversation at a time, they all slowed down. It was nearly impossible to describe what cancer-brain was like, so instead, I communicated how I felt. I was anxious, frustrated, forgetful, slow, sad and easily confused. With those pieces of knowledge, they had more of an understanding of where I was at. As they slowed down for me, I felt less anxiety to see my friends and be social, and social connections are so important for our well-being.

3. LOSS OF SPONTANEITY

I honestly could not count the number of people I've heard mention that they wish they could go back to "the way it was", how they "want the spontaneity back".

Sure, while you're fighting cancer, you're not suddenly ripping each other's clothes off in the television commercial break. But it's not just cancer that can change our intimate patterns. This is also normal for people in longer term relationships and anyone experiencing any stressful life-event. Also, let's think about when you were having spontaneous sex, what was happening in your life? Was there more time with each other? More foreplay? More flirting? More affection? More intimacy? Less stress?

Spontaneous sex is not the only type of sex. Removing spontaneity gives way for intention. Sure, a little more planning might not get your juices flowing in an instant, but it shows love, thoughtfulness and caring. That's pretty hot! You can make planned sex and intimacy special, like an upcoming and exciting date. It gives you time to prepare, to make sure you're well rested and not hurried or rushed. This allows you to get in the right headspace, which will guarantee you a better time. Plus, planning can be a lot of fun and is totally psychological foreplay.

A sexuality educator I was listening to recently, discussing this topic brought up this question and it was another one of those 'ahaaa' moments with me. They asked "how many romantic movies show the caring, intentional long-term portions of relationships where couples spend their day 'doing life'. A film where they cook, do the dishes and crash in bed late at night exhausted after a full day's work?" I'm going to say, hardly any.

Romantic films usually show the first stages, meeting, dating, flirting, the new relationship energy, the excitement and adrenaline, and when you have time for so much fun. Life isn't always like that, but that doesn't mean you can't connect and have pleasure.

Sex can still be fun, pleasurable and connective, even if it needs a bit of planning.

4. WHY LIBIDO DROPS

The two things I hear the most:

"I just don't want it anymore"

"It's like living with a friend"

I've been there and I am there. As I write this, the endocrine treatments I'm on have fizzled away the hormones that 'drive my drive' so to speak. It's tough, but it's not the end. Here I want to discuss how desire and intimacy work in the human body and the reasons we can experience drops in libido.

Here's the thing, desire/libido have a few layers to them. There's the physiological side, the psychological side and the neurological side. All of which can impact our libido.

The physiological side relates to the hormonal, physical and chemical changes in our body that treatments cause. That could be chemotherapy, medications, hormone treatments and others, which cause things like pain, dryness, changes in erection, fatigue and more. The psychological side relates to our emotions, patterns and stress. Both have an impact on our desire, and some are easier worked on than others.

The neurological side relates to how our brain is wired around what we do day to day, how we're feeling day to day / month to month, and influences how our brain is wired around things like libido. I discuss this in more depth in Part 2, but these three core aspects of ourselves (physiological, psychological & neurological) all impact our desire, the wanting.

It can be difficult to increase desire physiologically if we are still undergoing treatments such as hormone therapies, which impacts the way our body naturally works, like pushing a boulder up a hill. But that's not the end of it. If we're still on treatments and getting our 'drive' back to what it was isn't possible, there are still a few things that can be done to at least *improve* your desire (more on that later).

The psychological side is just as important, if not *more* important than the physiological. Did you know that stress impacts 100% of all human sexuality? 100%! A teeny tiny portion experience an increase in desire from stress, but most (I'm talking over 95% here) experience a drop in libido. And what's more stressful than cancer?

When we're stressed, we have less desire…when we have less desire, we're stressed. It's such a catch as the guilt and concerns about not wanting sex are contributors to us not wanting it.

But wait, there's more.

Our brain is our main sex organ. It's what's in between our ears, not our legs, that is our sex. And, as we all know, there are a lot of emotions and feelings that can occur in the back of our minds 24/7 and also play a large part in blocking our desire, 24/7.

Other than stress, another huge barrier to our wanting, is a sense of obligation or pressure that we *should* be wanting. I'll rephrase that. When we're tired, worried, stressed (even with a pre-cancer body), or forcing ourselves (I call it the 'should-brain'), our desire and libido drop, the 'wanting' just disappears. You're not going to want something that is an obligation. You're not going to want something that causes you emotional strain.

Just a few psychological barriers to your libido.

- Shame for not wanting sex.
- Stress or anxiety for experiencing changes in your sexuality.
- Guilt for asking a partner for sex.
- Guilt for saying no.
- Regret for saying yes.
- Awkwardness and distance as you don't want to 'hassle' your partner for affection.
- Stress & fear of living post diagnosis & recurrence.
- A sense of obligation and expectation that you should be sexual and having regular sex.
- Fear of hurting your partner.

- Financial and work stressors.

- Grief and loss for the way your body used to function.

- Feeling like you should be providing your partner with their needs (by the way, if your partner is desperate for sex, they can have sex with themselves, any time. Sex is never anything that is 'owed' to anyone).

- Feeling like you *should* be more sexual.

- Discomfort and stress as you don't know how to talk about things with your lover/partner.

- Anxiety/self-consciousness of your new body.

And so, so much more.

The core lesson I want you to understand from this, is that libido is extremely complicated and multi-layered. There is no quick magic-pill fix for our desire. I'm sorry if this is all doom and gloom right now, but I do have hope for you. Through understanding how our libido is affected on these levels, we can then work on rehabilitating it. And yes, you can (been there and done that), which I discuss in part 2 of this book and also guide people through in my online course.

5. TOUCHING ON TOUCH

Remember that cuddle hormone oxytocin that is released into the human body during sex, but also from other intimate forms of touch like cuddling? This hormone proves that touch is sex!

Not only is pleasure pleasurable, it's also connective. Feeling good with someone, touching them, having happy chemicals released into your body, it's a wonderful experience. Skin on skin contact, hugs, snuggles, hand holding, a good-night kiss together in bed. It's so easy to step away from affectionate touch as during cancer treatments, our bodies can feel strange, different and even foreign. Remind your body, remind your brain, touch can be enjoyable. Go slow, have a touch date with your partner/lover/yourself or date, and enjoy sensations for the sake of pleasure being pleasurable.

Think about it. We use cuddles to comfort upset children. Petting animals is good for our mental health. Loving touch contributes to our well-being and when it's absent, things can feel pretty lousy. When we feel more connected to our loved ones and ourselves, our nervous systems down-regulate (relax), and that allows us to feel safe and relaxed overall. Touch is the stepping stone towards your intimacy recovery.

6. COMMUNICATING IS HARD, BUT IT'S IMPORTANT

Please don't be down on yourself if you're struggling (whether you're a partner or the person diagnosed). Things are hard, things are different. It's okay, there are workarounds (which I'll get into soon). Ignore external pressures and expectations and focus on yourself and each other. Not only do our bodies and lives change from cancer, so do our roles. From lover to carer, friend to carer, partner to patient. You can get through it, together.

Silence is the enemy and can be common when we're finding things difficult. Fear and uncertainty are prevalent during treatments and we can withdraw from each other intentionally or unintentionally. It makes sense that we don't talk about the thing that's hard to talk about!

Fear of dating, meeting new people, of hurting a partner, not knowing how their/your new body works or not wanting to cause pain can all be reasons someone withdraws. Plus, your partner/loved one has seen you go through one of the hardest things of your life, be more unwell than ever, it's scary stuff.

For reasons above and more, not knowing how to interact and pulling away is common.

And for the people with the diagnosis, understanding what

is happening in our body and communicating that? That can feel impossible. Either way, humans have not evolved to read minds, so you'll need to break the silence and share what's happening. So often, the concerns we have in our minds seem a lot bigger when they stay in our minds. Talking is key.

And while we're at it, please don't compare yourself to anyone else or any other couples/people. It's the fastest way to unhappiness at any level and that includes comparing yourself to yourself, the 'pre-cancer you'. I call myself 'Tess BC' (BC = before cancer) when I'm in that loop. I often think of my pre-cancer body and mind, how I used to have less pain, more energy, body parts that used to be there, how I could remember things and focus on tasks, so you're not alone in this. I constantly remind myself, comparisons to others or the way things used to be won't change anything. It's such an easy pattern to fall into. I'm sorry to be so blunt as it's hard not to think about what has changed and how things used to be, but please try to think ahead. Cancer is different for everyone and every relationship is different.

There are millions of us fighting cancer, with suffering sexuality. It can be scary, but you don't have to do this alone.

Who to ask and how to ask

Communication with your loved ones isn't the only thing that's essential, but also communication with your treating team.

Knowing who to ask about sexuality, positioning, care & *safety* is something most of us don't know.

Here's a general summary.

Gynaecologists work with people who have a vulva and/or vagina. Urologists work with those who have a penis. Gastroenterologists and colorectal surgeons work with the digestive system including bowel cancers. Haematologists work with blood and lymphatic cancers. You will also have medical professionals relative to your treatments such as a radiation oncologist for radiotherapy treatments, an endocrinologist for hormone treatments and the effects they have on our bodies and sexuality, and your oncologist who oversees your treatments. You will have a surgical team relative to the type of procedure you will be having. Psychiatrists are who to speak with regarding mental health and medications, including which medications have which impacts on your sexuality.

All of these people plus your nurses, your doctor or GP (general practitioner if you're in Australia) are all trained to answer your questions.

There are also people like me (OTs) who focus on sexuality, there's pelvic floor physiotherapists and OTs, there are sexologists and sex counsellors as well. You will need to ask; you will need to be your own advocate for your sexuality. But don't worry, if they're not sure how to best answer your question, they will find someone who is. Your care is their priority.

I hear you saying "sure Tess, it's easy to tell us to ask medical professionals questions, but *how* do you ask the questions?" The first step (asking) is the hardest.... But you can do it, I've got your back!

How to say it out loud.

- "What are the precautions I need to take regarding sexual activities during this treatment?"
- "Do I need to avoid sex or do specific things safety-wise? If so, when and for how long?"
- "What do I and my partner/s need to know or do regarding intimate activities?"
- "I'd like to ask a few questions about sex and intimacy during my treatment. Is there a more private space we could go to?"
- "Is there someone I can speak with, who can answer questions about sex during and after treatment?"
- "We/I would like to discuss intimacy during/after treatment. Can we organise a time? And with who?"
- "I'm experiencing some changes with my (insert issue here). Who is the best person to speak to?"
- "How will this treatment affect me/us intimately?"

- "How long after surgery should we wait until it's okay to have sex again? And are there any positions or movements we should avoid?"

- "I'm not sure how to ask this, but I have some questions of a more private nature, who can I speak with about that?"

- "What are the precautions I need to take regarding sexual activities during chemo?"

- "Do I need to avoid sex or do specific things safety-wise during this treatment? If so, when and for how long after the infusion/procedure?"

If a healthcare professional isn't sure or cannot answer your question?

- "Thanks for letting me know, can you please ask someone who might be able to answer?"

- "Okay, can you please tell me who I can ask?"

7. FOR MY FELLOW RAINBOW-FLAGGERS

For people in the LGBTQIA+ community, medical institutions can be very difficult. I remember sitting in the chemo-chair with my then partner holding my hand. The nurse approached and looked at us holding hands, then looking at her said "oh, isn't that sweet you're such good *friends*". I know the nurse meant well, but it was devaluing to me and my partner. I did not feel like I was seen as a person, nor my partner respected. I also did not have the energy to continually educate everyone around me all day every day and advocate for who I am and for others. It's exhausting and with cancer, I didn't have it in me. So, I withdrew and I became reluctant to share my personal story with most clinicians. This is particularly important for people with cancers such as prostate, testicular, cervix, ovaries or breast (just to name a few), as these cancers are *very* gendered. Due to this people can isolate themselves from the supports that are out there as they may feel unwelcome or unseen. Speaking personally, the 'sisterhood' is very strong in breast cancer and as a non-binary person, was difficult to ignore. I avoided so many (pretty much all) support networks due to this as I did not feel welcome. If you're someone who resonates with this, if you belong to communities that are marginalised, I ask you to reach out. Reach out to that one person on your treating team you can have an honest, non-shaming conversation with. Reach out to the nurse asking for any resources the hospital knows of that are accessible and inclusive. Reach out to a friend, to find a cancer support group near you or online that is gender aware, recognises pronouns, alternative relationship models, and partnerships that are not only heterosexual. They are out there, but you may need help finding them. Feeling safe and supported is everything.

Asexuality

For any and all asexual folks (known as 'aces') reading this, know this book is also for you. Connection, intimacy and affection can all exist and should all exist, even if sex doesn't. If you're asexual, there is a ton of helpful information in this book for you to recover your intimacy and connection with yourself and others. As you may be getting the idea here (I hope you are!) that this book is about sexuality, intimacy, connection and love, not only sex. So, you're in the right spot for your cancer and intimacy recovery. Of course, there may be sections in this book that aren't right for you, but every single person reading this will have sections that aren't right for them for various reasons. Again, this book is your manual to pick and choose what's right for you.

If you're reading this and thinking "huh? What's asexual?", let me oh-so-briefly (and ineloquently) explain.

Think of the letter 'a' like the English word 'not'. Like, a-symmetrical (not-symmetrical) or a-neurotypical (not-neurotypical). Asexuality refers to the many people out there who live their lives as everyone else, just without having sexual desires, sexual attraction or having 'the sex'. To note, it's not nearly that simple and is much more complex than that basic explanation as people live and experience their asexuality differently, person to person.

I have clients, friends, people I support and also people I've taught & facilitated who are asexual and some are dating, some are romantic, some have partners, are passionate, affectionate people, have deeply loving and intimate relationships just not the sex and the sexual attraction part, and others don't wish for partners.

You might be thinking, oh yeah, priests and people of specific faiths are asexual. Well, kind of, but not quite. Celibacy is something that is a part of your life. Asexuality is who you *are*, not what you do. It's an orientation just like some people *are* straight/heterosexual, some *are* gay, or *are* bisexual etc. The 'A' in the LGBTQIA+ is for the orientation of asexuality (and for some, A is also used for 'allies').

This is very, *very* important for me to say. If you're asexual, this book is still for you.

8. WHAT HAVE WE COVERED?

- Language and definitions that we can get mixed up, that are handy to have a clear understanding of.

- Why connection is so important and all the different wonderful ways we can connect with each other.

- Why things like spontaneity and libido can take a back-seat, and the barriers for them thriving such as physical and psychological challenges.

- Communication tools, who to ask and how to ask those unsaid questions.

- And I've acknowledged the marginalisation that can occur in the healthcare system, encouraging us all to find the right support.

PART 2: STRATEGIES FOR CONNECTION

Tess Devèze

Without even realising it, during chemo, radio, multiple surgery recoveries and endocrine treatments, I lost my connection to those around me. I switched off my desire to connect, to reach out. And not only that, but the people around me were being cautious. They weren't scared of me; they were scared of hurting me. It was a real eye opener when I saw what was happening, and that's when I really put my thinking hat on.

This section offers ways and means to connect with those around you such as your friends, family, carers and partners. Connection is vital to being human, such as social connections, being part of the community, loving connections with partners, friends and family. Connection is the difference between surviving and living.

Included in this section are some strategies to connect with those around you including specific activities that I've taught others and love to do myself.

In my cancer-bubble of symptom management, I wanted to hide from the world. However, I began to realise there are ways to still connect with people. I learnt how to voice what I needed at the time, I learnt how to plan ahead, even when things were changing every hour for me, I also learnt activities, games, methods and solutions to have quality time with people. During treatments your connection to the world can be lost, but here in Part 2, I'll share solutions to keep these connections alive.

What I cover in this section

- Tips for loved ones.

- Communicating when we're not in the mood.

- Strategies around body-image changes.

- Approaches for fatigue and pain management.

- How treatments can affect your sexuality including chemotherapy, radiotherapy and hormone treatments.

- Pleasure, libido and sensory recovery.

- Navigating the dating arena.

- Simple and fun activities for connecting.

By the end of Part 2, you will have an understanding of the varied ways we can connect and communicate with those around us, including why that is important. You will also have a number of activities ranging from the purely verbal to ones involving touch, to offer a variety of ways to have quality time with anyone in your life.

9. HOW TO CRACK THE COMMUNICATION CODE

I was called in by a supported living space to assist a client living with a brain injury. This person had very severe impacts on their cognition and was unable to do things like remember things minute to minute, or have insight (amongst many other things). He was voicing things to the staff members and other people living in the space about being aroused and horny, so the staff wanted me to come in and see how I could help influence things to be comfortable and safe for everyone.

The staff were amazing, supportive and gentle while still setting boundaries, saying things like "that isn't appropriate" and "that's a private matter". I had several sessions with this person, who is a total sweetie by the way, having conversations and learning about them. I was using words like 'private things in private places' and 'inappropriate vs appropriate' to see if I could influence change in his behaviours. As this person was unable to learn new information, I had to work with what he already knew. After several conversations, I eventually learnt that the client actually interpreted those words differently to how the staff and I did. To him, the word 'private' actually meant something that was coercive, sneaky, to be done alone with bad intentions.

Through getting to know the client more, I then switched to words he himself used; 'for yourself' and 'by yourself'. He immediately got it. Rather than being told what he was saying should be 'private' (a word that meant something different to him), we switched to using words he did understand, "you need to keep that to yourself".

For a person that has difficulties learning, remembering and taking on new information, I'd cracked the code. This may seem small to you, but when I left the facility that day, I literally did a happy dance on the street as the door locked behind me on my way out. And spoiler alert; The staff are now able to manage his behaviour with ease, using this phrase.

I'm sharing this to demonstrate how important words are and that language is a code. Cancer is a whole new language, yes, but your relationships also have their own language, you have your own code. You'll notice I've written sentence strings and language samples of how to say things out loud throughout this book. The samples mostly all say similar things, just in different structures and oh-so-slightly different ways. To clearly communicate with your loved ones, find the language that resonates with you, or that you use together, so you can be understood and connect. Pick and choose what words may work for you, show this book to your partner so they can see what words and ways of saying things do (or don't) work for them. Use these language samples to find your relationship language, to crack the code for your connection.

10. TIPS FOR LOVED ONES

Seeing a loved one go through cancer is tough, and so can knowing what to say or how to act. Whether you're a carer, friend, family member or partner, there are ways to offer connection without overstepping a line. And don't worry, we won't break!

I once saw a young person ask on a cancer support forum "how long after chemo until I can kiss my mother on the cheek?" This post shocked me and showed me how some of us could see someone having chemo as being 'poisonous', as being 'toxic' or 'harmful'. Yes, caution is (very) necessary and the medical team must tell you about all of the risks involved in all treatments. People undergoing chemo, surgeries, radiotherapy, we can be seen as easily hurt, fragile or dangerous, and rightly so. There are many side-effects of treatments, some of them are mental and some of them are physical. However, let's remember this: connection is always important, and even if someone's body and mind are changing, there are still ways to be there with someone.

I dive into the impacts of particular treatments soon; however, it can understandably be hard to know what to do. It's also normal, when seeing a loved one be so unwell, to want to avoid causing any other harm and through that, create physical distance. That might look like reducing touch and physical contact, or even like possible avoidance. If you're a partner, lover, friend or carer of someone during treatment, I implore you, I beg you, to offer them touch. Treatment is damaging and also detaching. We need the treatment, yes, but we also need care, to feel connected to ourselves and to those around us. Don't be afraid of us, be cautious and curious with us. Think of it as getting into 'ask first' mode.

For simple touch, a peck on the lips or cheek? It's okay! We are not radioactive, we won't give you cancer and we won't break, if we all just take a little care. How do we know what to do or what not to do? We ask.

How to say it out loud.

- "Would you like me to take your hand?"
- "Is there any way you might like some loving/comforting touch right now?"
- "Would you like a hug?"
- "I'd love a cuddle; how does that sound to you?"
- "I'd love to connect with you, are there any sore spots I should avoid if I went in for a cuddle?"
- "I'd love to connect with you right now, is there a form of touch you would like?" (Arm around the shoulder, hand holding, hug from behind, foot massage and more.)
- "I love you and want to offer you connection, is there

anything that would comfort you at the moment?"

- "I miss you, but I'm worried I'll hurt you if I squeeze you too hard. Is there a way I can snuggle into you?"

- "I'm wanting to show you love and affection, such as a kiss on the lips or cheek, how do you feel about that?"

- I'm checking you out right now, fancy a kiss?

If you're being made an offer of connection and it's not a good time? I offer some examples shortly on ways to navigate that, however a simple, "thank you, but I'm not quite up for it at the moment" is perfect. Even if the person receiving this offer is not up for it right then, you're showing love, care, concern for their well-being and the desire to remain connected. It means the world.

Not in the mood?

Whether you're the person with cancer or the partner of, there will be times when you don't feel like being intimate with others, that is fine, that is normal, that is understandable. There will also be times when you feel like connecting somehow, but aren't sure how. There are lots of places to start: Get in the bath and relax or wrap yourself in blankets with a hot-water bottle, maybe touch your body, snuggle a pet with your favourite film, ask the person you're with to intertwine your legs while you both sit on the couch or lean into their chest.

During treatments, you're not going to want intimacy or touch all of the time, so feel free to let loved ones know how you're feeling and speak up in the moments it seems plausible. If you do receive an offer of intimacy and connection and you're not up for it? Remember, that's okay, that's fine, that's normal. But also remember to say thanks for the offer and be kind when you say no thanks, because you want the offers to keep coming!

How to say it out loud.

- "Thank you, that sounds amazing, it's not the best moment, can we see how I'm going later?" (Or tomorrow, or after lunch)
- "Thanks, I'm feeling quite nauseous/tired/some pain, for the moment I need to sit still, can we maybe connect later or another day?"
- "I'm really not feeling well, I'd like to sit alone for a while. Thank you so much for offering a cuddle, rain-check?"
- "I'd love to kiss you, but my mouth is a bit sore at the moment, would you like some soft neck touch instead?"
- "I'd love a hug, thank you, could you be careful around my arm? It's a bit sore."
- "I don't think I'm up for a hug right now, would you like to hold my hand?"

- "I'm pretty low on energy at the moment, but something soft and gentle would be lovely, like a snuggle?"
- Or if you're ADHD and ridiculously blunt like me "Thanks for the offer of a kiss, I'm currently trying not to vomit in my mouth, so will need to rain-check" (we both had a giggle at that).

To those undergoing treatments, if you feel your partner/lover/friend is avoiding you, unattracted to you and doesn't want to touch you? They may just be thinking they are protecting you, avoiding potentially hurting you or feel like they're pestering/pressuring you, so are pulling away. Be the one to communicate and offer a connection. Offer to snuggle, offer to touch their back while they're standing next to you, ask for a long hug hello, it guides them, and can lead to further connections. It meant the world to me, having my hand held and legs entwined on the couch with a cup of tea and chats. It was meaningful and intimate, that at times was my sex. Simple things like that were so important, and I know is/was to others during treatments.

11. BODY CHANGES & RECLAIMING CONFIDENCE

There are so many side-effects during treatments like fatigue, low mood, erection changes, and vaginal dryness. But there's also the visible effects such as loss of hair, weight changes, removed and/or replaced body parts and surgery scars. All can impact our physical appearance and the way we see ourselves.

As I write this, I have a surgery scar so large on my lower back I call it the 'shark-bite'. I have no nipple, just flat skin on a reconstructed breast that points in a different direction and is firm to touch. I have no sensation on that side of my chest, nor will I ever. I have stretch marks from weight gain and weight loss, I have patchy skin and my body doesn't function the way it used to. Here's the thing. People offer me compliments, but because I don't like my body, I simply don't believe them. You could tell me I'm beautiful a thousand times a day and it would be water off a duck's back. The changes to our body change the way we see ourselves which then influences the way we *feel* about ourselves. Because I don't believe you, I *won't* believe you.

The way towards us starting to believe the truth (that we are beautiful) is to create a shift in how we feel about ourselves. So, here's 10 ways to kick-start that process.

1. Switch.

Avoid marketing and media which is designed to make us feel ugly so we buy their products. What marketing tells us we should think 'beautiful' is, is completely unachievable and unrealistic for most humans (hence the gazillion dollar 'beauty industry'). Throughout our lives we're constantly told we're not beautiful enough, that we're not good enough, so we buy the things we're told will help. It's awful, it's everywhere and it can cause or contribute to poor mental health such as depression and anxiety. Take a look at the social media, magazines, even the TV shows you watch / are exposed to, and see if you can shift towards things that have realistic and un-shaming portrayals of human diversity and human beauty. Ask around, it's out there.

2. Health.

Eat well & Exercise. I know, it's so hard (especially on treatments), but you want to feel good in yourself and getting movement day to day and eating better can help us achieve that. It can be tough, but you've faced cancer, you can do anything. Even starting with 10 minutes of walking a day, switching a few sugar snacks with healthier ones or trying non-alcoholic beer/wine. Baby-steps.

3. Clothes.

Wear clothing that *feels* good. If you can't wear your old clothes anymore, put them away and get new ones. If fashion is meaningful to you, it's worth the investment. And watch out for behaviour changes. If buying a new wardrobe is not affordable, alternative options are second-hand/thrift stores, websites where you can hire clothing for those dressy occasions, or find friends with a similar body shape you can borrow off (or even get hand-me-downs from!).

If you find yourself dressing differently (baggier clothes, plain darker colours to not draw attention to yourself) or even not wanting to go to social events that may have an expectation of dressing up, this may indicate you're experiencing changes in the way you see yourself. Finding a few items of clothing that *feel* nice on your skin and boost your confidence, are worth their weight in gold.

4. Photos.

Remove photos and reminders of your pre-cancer body & replace them with *new* ones. Take some updated lovely photos of yourself or have someone else (a friend or photographer) help out, and update your social media and pop them around your home. Having constant reminders of who we were and what we've lost can get in the way of us processing and moving forwards. On dating apps? Update your profile with the new you, using these photos.

5. Quality connections.

Surround yourself with people you can communicate with honestly, that are positive in your life. This is over-simplifying it, but if people bring you down? Don't give them your time. You want relationships with people who contribute to you feeling comfortable, safe and respected. People you can share openly with, to feel supported and loved. Not sure how to know? Notice how you feel after you've spent time with or spoken with people. Do you feel good? Heard? Supported? Or do you notice with some people you walk away feeling drained, misunderstood or judged? Noticing how you feel is a powerful indicator to who you want to spend time with.

6. Treats.

Treat yourself by doing things that help you feel good (helping others, dressing up, exercise, getting a massage, self-pleasure, a bath). You want to experience more 'feeling good' and have that feeling in your life more.

7. Touch.

Connect, have affection, have kisses and skin on skin contact. Hug your friends, hold hands, kiss your partner for the sake of it. Slowly get used to your new body together with a partner and be open about your feelings. If you're with a partner or on a date and feeling shy or you're not sure where to start, play the 2-minute game (detailed in the upcoming section 'simple ideas for connecting'). Touch and intimacy contribute to our mental health and well-being, plus our confidence and self-esteem.

8. Embrace your shy.

You don't have to be naked, or full-frontal to have sex. You can be intimate with clothes on, lights-off / low or have sex in positions where you're not face to face which I cover in the 'sexual positions, techniques and tools' section later in Part 3. There are ways. Fear of getting naked in front of a lover/partner/date is common. Think about it, if we're not feeling great about our bodies, it makes sense we feel others won't also.

9. Grieve.

Give yourself time to grieve. This is loss. Loss of who we were, and it's okay that you're sad. Allow yourself time to process and be kind to yourself. We lose so much, and we can't move on until we can comfortably say goodbye. It's natural for you to find it difficult to love a different you, but if you find your grief interfering with your life and relationships? Please seek support from a counsellor or psychologist. You don't have to do it alone.

<u>10. Words.</u>

Ask your partner/friends for compliments, but on WHO YOU ARE, *not* how you look. Why? Because if we don't agree, we simply won't agree. Being complimented on you as a person rather than physical appearance is much more believable, and is the stepping stone towards feeling more confident. And while we're at it, you can ask for compliments in those moments of insecurity. This may seem forced and construed, but it doesn't mean that a compliment is false just because you've reminded someone you would like to hear one. You're just giving someone permission to offer you flattery in a situation where they may be scared to comment on your appearance or person in any way. It's easier than you think, here's some examples:

How to say it out loud; asking for compliments.

- "I'm feeling a bit low, I'd welcome compliments at the moment."
- "I'm not feeling great, hearing nice things about me might help."
- "I'm feeling pretty self-conscious about my appearance, thoughts?"
- "I'm embarrassed to go out, I feel like I look sick, do I look okay?"

Giving compliments without the beauty focus.

- "I love seeing you smile; it makes me happy."
- "I think you did really well today in conversation."
- "Hearing you laugh gave me so much joy, I think you're amazing."
- "I love you."
- "Everyone was so happy to see you today, you mean a lot to your family/friends/colleagues."
- "I'm so glad you're in my life."
- "You look great in that colour."
- "I love what you're wearing."
- "You're such a great friend."
- "I love our friendship/relationship/connection."
- "You did great today, everyone seemed so happy to see you."
- "You look happy today."
- "Your eyes are shining."
- "You look sexy in those pants."
- "I'm perving on your arse right now, do you mind?"

It isn't a cure, but a little love goes a long way!

12. MANAGING FATIGUE

I was that person who thought that the word 'fatigue' was like when you've been the tiredest you've ever been in your life. I was so, so wrong! I couldn't comprehend the severity of what fatigue really was (until chemo and every treatment following).

I suffered severe fatigue and still do. For some people, fatigue is something that can last years after treatments and like everything else in cancer, affects us differently. My body likes to jump into 5–9-day migraines when I push myself beyond my energy levels (things like going to the supermarket without having rested beforehand or seeing more than 2 clients in a day can push me over the edge). It makes sense when we are fatigued, sex and intimacy can seem unachievable.

Fatigue is lingering and is an invisible symptom. I can hear the voices of so many of my clients (and myself) saying those words "I'm just so tired", "I have no energy". However, fatigue and energy levels can be *somewhat* managed.

Energy conservation and fatigue management are things OTs receive clinical training in, and honestly, is a whole book unto itself. So, here's just a few tips.

<u>A fatigue diary.</u>

Keep a fatigue diary, note the times in the day you have more or less energy. Are there some activities that really wipe you out? (Like cleaning). Or some that give you a little extra bounce? (Like light exercise). Write down when you have the energy to make a sandwich, go for a short walk, were too tired to leave the bed for several hours or felt okay to try and be social. You want to find a pattern, to find those energy 'sweet spots' during your days or weeks. Are there activities that you notice increase your fatigue a lot? Plan them at times when you have a moment to rest afterwards. Are there times in your day where you have more energy? That's when you want to organise some intimate times. Get the supermarket to deliver the food to your home and get cuddly with your partner instead.

Planning around fatigue.

You can also look at what you do day to day, and arrange your activities so you can have the more demanding tasks, split up throughout the day, with the more low-key tasks between. Maybe you do some work, rest, then go for a walk to help your energy out, then have some yummy time with your partner when they get home from work, get dinner delivered and rest, then clean up before bed. Alternating high energy tasks with lower energy tasks can be very useful to get through the day.

Below is an example of what a client and I came up with, to spread out their demanding tasks. They were self-employed and of course, your life will be completely different to this. But I hope it gives you an idea of ways to break up activities and have rest breaks. Even if it's only one or two days of the week this type of scheduling is possible, or switching around only a few daily tasks in your week, it's better than nothing. Anything is better than nothing!

Time of day	Activity	Energy level
0800	Shower & dress	Uses energy
0830	Breakfast, have meds, watch the news (seated)	Resting
0900	Computer work	Uses energy
1000	See a client	Uses energy
1115	Rest in chair, while doing computer admin on laptop	Resting
1200	Make & eat lunch	Uses energy
1245	Phone a friend/family, lying down/seated in chair	Resting
1300	Go to an appointment/see another client	Uses energy
1430	Light exercise	Creates energy
1500	Get groceries delivered, continue work/see a client	Uses energy
1730	Solo-pleasure/partnered-pleasure time & rest	Can create energy!

1830	Dinner (cook/get delivered)	Uses energy
1930	Rest & digest, & get couch snuggly	Resting
2100	Tidy up kitchen, maybe prep breakfast for tomorrow?	Uses energy
2130	Go to bed, maybe more rest: reading/TV.	Resting

Notice how the time for intimacy and connection was early evening? The assumption that we need to be intimate at the end of the day is ludicrous, as that's generally when we're at our tiredest. Personally, when I plan a date with a partner, it's late afternoon and we get intimate *before* dinner. After dinner I turn into a slug, and pretty much all activities are too much for me. Again, we're all different which is why a fatigue diary is so important. Tracking your days, your activities and your energy levels gives you the information you need to conserve energy and, to connect. This goes for partners too, it's important for everyone to take a look at your schedules and brainstorm ways to make daily life more enjoyable and a little easier.

Here's another example. I was having a session with a couple navigating a stage 4 diagnosis. Fatigue and energy to connect was their main concern at the time. We talked about their schedules, her fatigue patterns and their working schedules. He worked *very* long hours during the week so they didn't get much quality time together on weekdays. He was s spritely morning person and woke up early on weekends. Due to treatments, she slept longer hours and had more energy later in the mornings after she woke up. Through some brain-storming, we realised that if he delayed his Saturday morning bike ride by a few hours, they would have quality time together when she woke up a few hours after he did. We even brain-stormed what he could do at home, for the few hours he was awake and she wasn't instead of riding (like coffee and a crossword, reading, gardening etc.). Once she woke up and they had some intimate time together, she could rest and he could go for his ride. They both were still able get the sleep they needed and do the activities that were meaningful to them, including having intentional time to be together. If you're partnered, think of this as a collaboration. Your relationship is worth it, your connection is worth it!

Exercise.

I'll be honest. I *hate* the fact that exercise is good for you. Why can't eating deep-fried chicken in bed while watching Star Trek be good for our bodies? What's even worse than the fact that exercise is good for us, is that exercise can give us *more* energy. It was almost upsetting that every time I got back from my daily walks during chemo, I felt better. Every time, guaranteed. Have caution here, yes, exercising can increase your energy levels, but you don't want to push yourself too hard, or you'll go backwards fatigue wise. It's a delicate dance to find what's right for you. If you can access an exercise physiologist (ask your treating hospital for an appointment or your doctor to give you a community referral), they can assess your current level of physicality and give you an individual exercise regime. Don't worry, it won't be an hour at the gym every day, maybe a short gentle walk each day, but better to follow the recommendations of a professional who knows you and your situation.

If walking isn't appealing to you at all, yoga is another option which is amazing for our bodies and energy levels. Something that got me through chemo and I still do regularly for my fatigue is yoga. But for me, I'd never do it if I had to get to a class as it's just too much effort for me. So, I do it online with a wonderful person who has a YouTube channel called 'Yoga With Adriene'. She offers free yoga programs and classes, of all levels and they're pretty great.

I'm sorry to say it again, but it's so important, gentle exercise is really great for your mental health, your body and your energy levels.

Perhaps you're thinking, "but Tess, sometimes my energy

levels don't follow a predictable pattern". Good point, I have an idea for you.

Predicting around the unpredictable.

Around the fluctuating and low energy levels treatments can cause, there are forms of connection, intimacy and play that can still connect you with others. The key is to know your options, discuss them, see where you're at and do what you think is manageable, for where you're at. What I'm not going to recommend is 'winging it'. Things don't always work out how we want them to and that is a part of life, not just with cancer treatments in the mix. Have a few options up your sleeve. When you set a date or catch up with someone, suggest 3 options which vary in energy levels and confirm which one you'd like to do depending on how you're feeling, *on the day.*

As an example, say you're wanting to see a close friend. You could discuss a few options such as:

- If you have more energy: Having a lovely meal at a local restaurant to treat yourselves.

- If you have less energy: Have your friend over and they can cook while you chat and spend time together.

- Even less energy: If conversation seems a bit daunting, but you still want to connect, your friend can bring food over and you get comfy on the couch and watch a film together.

Another example of three suggestions you could 'pencil in' that might suit varied levels of energy if you're wanting some connective time with a partner/lover are:

- Go for a nice dinner or lunch at one of your favourite places (all reservations can be cancelled if need be).

- If going out isn't possible, play the two-minute game (detailed soon in 'simple ideas for connecting') at home and have food delivered.

- Have a bath together or a snuggle and play Q&A (also described in the abovementioned section).

Given the challenges of treatments, the best thing is to plan those times where connection is possible. This could be well in advance, such as those times when your fatigue and pain may be at its lowest in your days or weeks. Unfortunately, as much as you plan ahead, you can never guarantee how you will feel. It's vital those around you understand you may need to cancel or change plans as well as having a few options up your sleeve. And hey, if trying to plan these things seems like too much effort? Show this section of the book to your loved ones or friends and they can do the planning for you.

13. MANAGING PAIN

Pain is extremely complex and has many forms, be it chronic, neurological, musculoskeletal and more. This section is in reference to people experiencing pain from treatments and is very general. Your treating team is there to help you with your pain, specific to your body and medical history. For people who have pre-existing neurological conditions, past injury, chronic illness, trauma or are living with disability, pain may have been a part of your life well before treatments. If you're someone experiencing pain from treatments and have pre-existing conditions, please chat to your treating team. In particular, your oncologist, doctor, physiotherapist or OT who may be able to connect you with a pain clinic.

Regarding pain experienced from treatments, side effects can persist and our body can take time to heal. We may experience pain from surgeries, radiotherapy, bone pain from endocrine treatments, nerve pain from chemo and more, in many different ways.

You know the saying "no pain, no gain?" We're often given the message that if we want to make progress that it's going to have to hurt. While this can be true at the gym (depending on how you work out), this concept doesn't belong in sex and intimacy.

I once heard a sexuality educator say "no pain, *no pain*" and

I instantly loved it. Sex and intimacy shouldn't ever be painful. Pain is our body's alarm system to let us know something isn't quite right, its useful information, so don't push through it. It won't be pleasurable and it's not going to contribute to you wanting to go back for more. In fact, it could have the opposite effect and put you off. Sex and intimate touch should *never* cause pain, regardless if you have an illness you're dealing with or not. Whatever your age, gender, health status, orientation or pleasures, you should never experience pain during sex and if you do, you should stop. If you do experience painful penetration, or have genital pain, it can be frustrating but know that it's common and is often overcome. If it's painful or sore, and you don't stop, it could cause damage to already sensitive tissues. Remember, 'no pain, *no pain*'. Be gentle with yourself, there are plenty of ways to connect.

Planning around pain.

I found that it was best to plan to have connection when I felt the most well, and was experiencing the least pain during my days and weeks. So, just like your fatigue diary, try to track your pain with a calendar or diary also. Look for the patterns to find times when pain is lower or is absent, or maybe when your painkillers take best effect so you can plan for connection around those times. My pain was very unpredictable in its varied forms, however by keeping a record and flicking through my notes, I did find patterns which enabled me to predict when I would be experiencing less pain in my routine. After exercise was when my pain was lower, also, during chemo, I was able to predict the days when my migraines would start and end. Seeing I would be very unwell for 8-10 days helped me schedule something before I was 'clocking off' into what I then called my 'migraine-holes'. It also gave me something to look forward to, a lovely lunch with a friend, a partner coming over or some massage swaps after my migraines subsided. I needed those little lights at the end of each daily tunnel.

Alternatives.

From tracking your pain in a diary, you may notice a few themes, such as things that can cause a flare-up or more pain. Common ones are things like housework, buying groceries, or not having rest breaks throughout the day. Just like in the fatigue section how I suggested you break up your daily activities with restful tasks in between, it can be very helpful to do the same regarding pain. Spacing out the tasks which take a toll on your body, so you can rest in between or time them around your pain meds can be a game changer. For an example of what that could look like, refer to the daily schedule example in the 'fatigue' section.

You can also find alternatives, shortcuts and life-hacks

depending on what you find causes you pain. If vacuuming causes a flare-up, can you or a friend gift you a robo-vac? If buying and carrying groceries is too much, can you get them delivered or order online? If standing to cook increases pain, can you sit on a stool in the kitchen while chopping veggies, or do a bulk cook on Sundays so you can reheat meals during the week? Can a friend come over and help you with that? Maybe sitting at a desk for too long causes pain, so set an alarm every 30-40 minutes so you can regularly stretch and move your body. These may seem small, but finding these little life-shortcuts can offer relief and reduce flare-ups to give you more capacity for the good things, like intimacy and connection.

<u>Relaxation.</u>

Anticipation, anxiety and stress around intimacy can cause our muscles to become tense and this can increase or contribute to pain. Try to relax. Go slowly. Explore your body alone, use touch, slowly gauge your body and its responses. If you're planning sex, have a nice bath beforehand or warm up with a massage first. It's better to take more time and experience more enjoyment, than to push yourself and have a shorter, less enjoyable time.

<u>Warmth.</u>

Joint and muscle pain can cause discomfort and really got in the way of my wanting to connect with those around me. I found that warmth really helped me. Having a warm shower or bath can help relax your muscles and ease joint pain as it creates blood flow. Just make sure you always have water within arm's reach, as dehydration can exacerbate pain! If you want to engage in self/solo-sex, pleasuring yourself in the bath is ideal if you can get comfortable. Your body is warm and relaxed, two key elements that help with experiencing pleasure.

Don't have a bath? Get your hands on an 'electric throw', a blanket that is heated and you can lie on it or under it during intimate activities. Or warm the bed in advance with an electric blanket or hot water bottle. With a little planning and prep, things can be easier.

Experiment with positions.

If you have pain, alternative positions can be explored or using cushions to support joints or change pelvic angles. Where there is a will, there is usually a way! Keep a sense of humour and exploration about it and know that what worked last time might not work the next time. Refer to the 'sexual positions' section in part 3 of this book for specific examples.

Go slow and communicate.

It's essential when you're exploring ways to engage intimately and you have any type of pain, to go slowly and communicate.

Stop any activity that doesn't feel right. It could be that you're not aroused enough yet, you may need to avoid certain movements for a while after surgery or it might be that you need to speak with a doctor to determine what is causing the pain and how to treat it. It's okay, there are options and it's worth remembering it may not be permanent.

It isn't spontaneous, but having a comfortable, more pleasurable connection is much more important than having a surprising one. And remember, talk to your medical treating team.

It's worth noting here, that the happy chemicals pleasure, arousal and orgasms release in our body can also relieve pain. I have many clients with chronic illness and disability who use pleasure as pain relief, so they can have moments in their life pain free. Just one more reason why pleasure is so healthy for us!

For those curious as to why I've left out the topic of vaginal pain and dryness out of this section, don't worry. I discuss this in depth in part 3 of this book (refer the section titled 'our poor vajootz').

14. CHEMOTHERAPY

I get asked about this topic a *lot*. The toxicity of chemotherapy is understandably of concern to those receiving it, but it's okay to be close, intimate and sexual with people on chemo, with a few precautions.

Yes, we need consider the toxicity of chemo, but there's other things too, such as low white blood cell counts increase risk of infections and pregnancies can have problems. You may need to wear barriers during sex, or use barriers for specific amounts of time before or after your infusion. By 'barriers' I mean safer sex items like condoms or dental dams (which I discuss more in part 3 in the section titled 'lube is life').

So, how do you know what precautions you need to follow during chemo? Ask! As your precautions will differ depending on what chemo type and regime you're on, you'll need to ask your treating team.

Who?
Your oncologist and chemotherapy nurse will 100% know the answer to your questions.

When?
Preferably before you start chemo, but it's never too late to ask (I had these discussions while I was sitting in the chemo chair).

Now here's something very important. If you're someone wanting to have penetrative sex during chemotherapy (vaginally or anally), lubricants are *essential*. Your body will be dehydrated and your tissues may become extra sensitive from this treatment. Lubricants are easily purchased and they really do make things better, however, please use something other than water-based lubricants. They get absorbed into your body like a sponge (as that's what the body does even when it's not dehydrated), so you need something that will stay slick for longer. I recommend silicone-based lubes Überlube or Sliquid Silver, they're so great. Others use organic coconut oil for lubrication (but can cause thrush with some people, so have caution), or an organic wax-based product Olive & Bee. Lubricants are to me, a safer sex item and worth proper discussion, so in part 3 of this book, I cover lubricants in much more detail.

If you experience pain during penetration and you're using lubricants, *stop* and chat with your treating team. For those with a vagina, you may need to use an internal moisturiser to help the tissues rehydrate and become less sensitive. Heal first, play later (refer to the 'our poor vajootz' section for more on this topic). Remember, no pain - no pain! Get it checked out.

Also, your sexual function may change, things may not work as they used to. Maybe your orgasms take longer, maybe they're more or less intense, maybe you don't orgasm anymore, perhaps your erections are changing, you no longer get wet or you simply want sex less. These are common side-effects from chemo and may not be permanent. Remember that your body is processing toxins to treat a disease. You will experience changes in your body, if you're worried, chat with your oncologist or doctor.

I was told before I started chemotherapy that I would need to wear protection to avoid causing my partner harm, as I would be so toxic. I was petrified of hurting the people around me, I honestly felt like I could harm the people I loved from how 'poisoned' I was. I was scared. I truly regret not asking my chemotherapy nurse for more information about what exactly I needed to be careful of and when. As it wasn't as bad as I thought and from that fear, I withdrew physically from the people around me. So, please learn from my mistakes and ask the nurses/the oncologist for clear guidance.

What do we do?

- Communicate with each other and your oncologist / chemo nurses.

- Be transparent about your side-effects such as pain, fatigue, rashes, changes in sensitivity, pleasure, libido. Tell your date/partner(s) what's going on and how you're doing. Sex can be soft, gentle, and doesn't need to involve penetration. If you're open about how you're doing and what's going on in your body, you can still be intimate around that.

- Use a silicone, wax or oil-based lubricant (see the 'lube is life' section in part 3 for more info).

- Explore touch that isn't penetration or orgasm focussed, like the two-minute game (see the 'simple ideas for connecting' section).

- Use barriers if/when needed as advised by your oncologist such as external/internal condoms or dental dams.

- You could shower before and after intimacy to help avoid UTIs.

- Remember, your body not acting normally during chemo is pretty normal!

- For partners: Be gentle, we won't break. Yes, we're sick, but you can totally touch us. Cuddle us, have sex with us, just check in, communicate and remember...don't be afraid of us, be cautious *with* us!

How to say it out loud.

- "What are the precautions I need to take regarding sexual activities during chemo?"

- "Do I need to avoid sex or do specific things safety-wise during chemo? If so, when in my cycle and for how long after the infusion?"

- "Do I need to do anything different sex-wise while I'm taking these chemo tablets?"

- "I'd like to ask a few questions about sex and intimacy during my treatment, is there a more private space we could go to?"

- "I have a few questions about having chemo and if that changes anything sexually, is there someone I can ask?"

- "My partner and I would like to discuss bedroom activities during treatment, can we organise a time? And with who?"

- "Can I have sex during chemotherapy?" (If yes) "Is there anything in particular I need to know regarding safety?"

- "If I do need to wait, how long do I need to wait until after my infusion / taking these tablets?"

- "Is there a resource where I can get this in writing? It's hard for me to remember details".

- "Can you please write this down for me? As I won't remember everything and this is important to know, thank you".

If a healthcare professional isn't sure or cannot answer your question?

- "Thanks for letting me know, can you please ask someone who might be able to answer?"

- "Okay, can you please tell me who I can ask?

15. RADIOTHERAPY

Much like every cancer treatment there is, radiation therapy is not one-size-fits-all, and is unique for each person. Plus, can be delivered in two primary categories, internally or externally (from inside the body or outside the body). My personal experiences with radiotherapy were external, I lay down with my arms above my head and they used a beam to target radiation on my body, including my chest, armpit and neck. I had daily sessions and over the 5-week period, my what I then called 'my bacon titty' became raw and sore. The pain was one thing, but the fatigue was another. I did not anticipate the levels of fatigue I experienced during radiotherapy, but looking back now it makes sense. We are being introduced to radiation and every day we are exposed to a little bit more. Our body uses energy to try and heal and every day as we're exposed to more, this ads to what our body has to process. So, it's logical our fatigue worsens as we progress through daily treatments. For strategies regarding intimacy around pain and fatigue, see the recent 'pain' & 'fatigue' sections and also in part 3 in the 'sexual positioning' section. There are other side-effects such as hair loss and nausea, and some can experience lowered libido. For more on that, take a look at the libido information in part 1 and also the 'pleasure is a bicep' section coming up.

People can receive internal radiation in varied ways for

various cancers such as cervical, pelvic, prostate, rectal, uterine and more. I know people who have received internal pelvic radiation and have a wide range of aftercare and impacts including dilator use. Dilators are objects of varying sizes that are inserted into the vaginal canal regularly, to maintain canal shape, size and function. Aftercare can vary from using internal creams and dilators for a few weeks after radiotherapy finishes, to using them over years and even permanently. I know some who include dilator use each morning in their shower routine, others who experience pain need to be slow and careful, so need to carve considerable time (and energy) out of their day. This can be an extremely difficult thing to manage and endure, and can hold a lot of trauma. Please have discussions with your radiation oncologist regarding the side-effects short and long term, relative to the treatment they recommend.

For people who have received internal radiation anally and rectally for cancers such as bowel, anal or rectal, similar impacts can be experienced as those who receive vaginal radiation. The internal canal can tighten, shrink or have changes in sensation. Although dilators are labelled to be used for vaginas, I do know of people who have also used them for their anus and rectal canal. Using them exactly as they are intended, starting with the smallest size, using a lot of lube and slowly over time increasing the dilator size, to shape the canal and help open it up. This of course, should not be done without consulting your treating team as you could do more damage than good if not done properly.

Also, penetrative sex may be painful after radiation, and for some who may have targeted radiation deeper inside the pelvis, say the cervix or the rectum, penetration can be painful deeper inside. There is an intimacy aid called the 'Ohnut', it's a wearable item which reduces the depth of penetration by shortening toys and penises. It's comfortable and is getting wonderful results, so if you're experiencing pain/discomfort deeper inside, this may be worth looking into.

It's very different for everyone depending on your particular cancer and treatment, so asking these questions beforehand can help you prepare psychologically and physically.

How to say it out loud.

- "You mention that the radiation will be delivered inside my body, how does that work?"

- "I'd like to ask a few questions about sex and intimacy during my treatment, is there a more private space we could go to?"

- "Will there be people in the room to support me during this process?"

- "What are the side-effects sexually after this treatment?"

- "Given my pelvis/genitals/anus/lower abdomen are

receiving radiation, will this affect my sexual function?"

- "I'm worried about the impacts this will have on my private life; can we talk about this in detail?"
- "After having internal radiation, is there a specific lubricant I should avoid/use during penetrative sex? Can you please be specific as to the type and brand I should use?"
- "Can this treatment impact my ability to get an erection?"
- "Will I be naked in front of many people?"
- "Can I have sex during this treatment? If so, are there any precautions I need to take? Why and for how long?"
- "Is this something that's going to interfere with me being able to have a child in the future?"
- "How long should we wait before trying to get pregnant after this treatment finishes?"
- "I'm really nervous, can we please go over this in detail again?
- "You mention dilator use, can you please give me some written information on them to take home with me?"
- "Can you please give me the name of a few support groups which focus on pelvic radiotherapy and dilator use?"
- "Are there specific timeframes we should wait before having sex after this treatment?"

- "Is there anything I can do to help prepare my body in advance?"

- "Is there some written information you can pass on that covers how this works and any side-effects?"

If a healthcare professional isn't sure or cannot answer your question?

- "Can you please find someone who could help me with this? I'm happy to wait."

- "Okay, can you please tell me the name and contact info of who I can ask?"

There are many various methods and regimes for radiation therapy and you will have an entire radiation therapy team who are there to answer your questions. It's never too late to ask.

16. HORMONE TREATMENTS

I've been undergoing endocrine treatments for just over 2 years now and I've 3 more to go and let me tell you this, it's *not* a walk in the park. I've really struggled with this treatment and so many others do. Our endocrine system is one of the most underrated and essential systems for our daily function. We all know about the cardiovascular system, with which our heart pumps blood throughout our body, or our nervous system, which is the control centre for our movement, sensation and organ function. But when we hear 'endocrine system' or 'hormones' so many of us shrug it off as non-essential to our day-to-day health. Our endocrine system is a very important mechanical cog in the well-oiled machine that is the human body. Hormones aren't just so we can develop sexually. The glands throughout our body that the endocrine system controls that release hormones into our body influence things like our metabolism, sleep, mood, growth, bone health and so, so much more.

There are cancers that love specific hormones and their presence helps the cancer grow, imagine it like a food source. Some cancers such as breast or uterine cancers love oestrogen. Other cancers like prostate, may be receptive to testosterone and one of the marvels of modern medicine is we can now use treatments to block certain hormones, which can help reduce the cancers size, slow its growth down and reduce risk of recurrence.

And of course, like everything in cancer, treatments vary person to person and can be administered by pills, injections, insertables and more. Altering the endocrine system by treatments, including surgeries which remove organs and glands that belong to it, can have very severe impacts on a person's life. Impacts that are mostly invisible and therefore, not recognised by those around us as serious, or real. I'm here to tell you they are very, very real and some of my darkest days during my cancer experience were due to the endocrine treatments I'm currently on.

My breast cancer loves oestrogen and progesterone, so at the age of 36 with the marvels of an abdominal injection each month, I was chemically induced (thrown) into menopause. This was a huge shock to my body, as I wasn't naturally strolling down the menopause path over a timeframe of years. No, I was thrown off the cliff into that menopause ocean and I didn't know how to swim. Thank the universe for my breast care nurses, my oncologist, my psychiatrist and my partners for helping me keep at it, to keep trying different medications and therapies to ease the side-effects. It took time (years), but I'm in a much better space than the absolute mess I was less than a year ago.

It's not just people with vulvas that suffer the impacts of

medically onset menopause. People born with testicular systems, who have penises and prostates can undergo the removal of testosterone via androgen deprivation therapy (ADT). They suffer the same effects on daily living (hot-flushes, sleep deprivation etc.), just as being thrown into menopause does.

Some impacts of endocrine treatments are:

Libido can drop with the sudden absence of certain hormones in our body, so take a look at the information on desire and libido in part 1 and in the next section titled 'pleasure is a bicep'.

We can experience genitourinary (genital and/or urinary tract) changes, lose erection (see the 'changes in erection' section in part 3), experience vaginal atrophy (see the section titled 'our poor vajootz' in part 3) and experience pain in our bones and joints (see the 'managing pain' section just gone). Then there's the 'brain-fog / cancer-brain' as some call it, which is actual cognitive dysfunction. I felt like I was watching myself experience Alzheimer's. I couldn't remember people's names, how to get to my local shops, sometimes I got lost and relied on the kindness of strangers to help me find my way home. It was scary and stressful.

As mentioned, I cover vaginal atrophy in depth in part 3, however the absence of certain hormones can also cause the vaginal canal to shorten/shrink, causing pain and discomfort. Penetrative sex could feel 'tighter' and also uncomfortable deeper inside if your vaginal canal is slightly shorter. The 'Ohnut', which I mentioned in the radiation therapy section works wonders. It is a comfortable silicone item worn on penises and toys, and is designed to reduce the 'depth' of penetration. It's a wonderful item and is worth looking into.

Sleep disruption is very common, so please take a look at the 'fatigue' section if you have not already. It's easy for me to brush this off as just another side-effect, but sleep deprivation is all encompassing and had me at breaking point several times. Due to night-sweats, brain-chatter and restless leg syndrome (you'd think I was running a marathon in my bed); I couldn't sleep. Sleep impacts our mood, our emotional resilience, our appetite, libido, our cognitive processes, how we think and our motivation. Talk to your treating team if you're experiencing sleep disruption as there are ways and means to help ease those dreaded nights. Especially if things like night-sweats and hot-flushes are keeping you awake. Your oncologist, endocrinologist, gynaecologist, urologist and personal doctor, will have support and suggestions. Sleep is everything and when I wasn't getting enough of it, was a major player in what I call my 'cancer-holes', the times when I was not able to cope.

There are also the psychological impacts from changes in our endocrine system, such as depression, anxiety, chronic stress and fear as we watch our body and mind seem almost out of control. Seeking support from a cancer-informed counsellor or psychologist can be your saving grace.

For people with a hormone receptive cancer diagnosis who are transgender, non-binary, gender non-conforming, intersex, someone who is or may be undertaking medical-gender-affirmation therapies that may (or may not) involve hormone treatments, it's very important you find a professional you can speak with openly. You want to be able to ask any and all questions you may have regarding treatments and you need to do that in a safe environment. Again, this could be a task for a friend, or a nurse to find the right clinician for you.

And if something doesn't feel right? It's likely because something isn't. It's important things like medications and your dosages are right for you so again, communication is everything and so is asking for follow-up appointments with your team.

How to say it out loud.

- "What are the side-effects sexually of this treatment?"
- "I'd like to ask a few questions about sex and intimacy during my treatment, is there a more private space we could go to?"
- "I'm worried about the impacts this will have on my private life; can we talk about this in detail?"

- "Can this treatment impact my ability to get an erection?"

- "I've heard vaginal pain is a side-effect, what does that actually mean?"

- "Is there a way I can prep in advance, to prevent vaginal dryness?"

- "Are there medication options that don't impact my sexuality?"

- "Can I have sex during this treatment? If so, are there any precautions I need to take? If not, why and for how long?"

- "Is this something that's going to interfere with me being able to have a child in the future?"

- "How long should we wait before trying to get pregnant after this treatment finishes?"

- "I'm really nervous, can we please go over this in detail again?"

- "Are these hormones going to change my physical appearance?"

- "Is there some written information you can pass on that covers how this works and any side-effects to expect?"

- "Is there someone I can talk too about if I can take these treatments while undergoing hormonal gender affirmation?"

- "Are these hormone treatments going to have side-effects

that might feminise or masculinise me?"

If a healthcare professional isn't sure or cannot answer your question?

- "Not a problem, I'm happy to wait while you find someone who can help".

- "Okay, if you could write down the name of the right person to talk to, or some clinical resources I can access that'd be great, thanks."

17. PLEASURE IS A BICEP (RECOVERING LIBIDO)

I'm Australian and I don't beat around the bush (Aussie slang for, I'm honest and to the point). I won't tip-toe around and fluff how hard this is. It's hard. I'm also here to give you hope.

Like a broken record, I mention that our brain is our largest sex organ and the best thing about it, is that it's not solid concrete, forever stuck in its ways. I've worked in neurological rehabilitation in public and private hospitals working with brain injury, stroke, spinal cord injury and more, so I'm going to do my best not to get carried away in my neuro-speak. But here's a vitally important piece of knowledge for your future relationship and life overall.

Your brain can *change*. It's called 'neuroplasticity' and those of us who work in the neurosciences have a saying, "*Use it or lose it*". What this means is that the more we do something, the 'larger' the sections in our brain get which are dedicated to that area / to doing that thing. It's like the more you exercise your bicep, the larger and stronger it gets. The same thing happens with our neural pathways and the sections in our brain that are dedicated to doing the thing or feeling the thing. Here's the interesting part, the opposite also happens, the 'lose it' in that motto.

If we don't do something often, just like that bicep would get weaker without regular use, the pathways or connections in our brain get 'smaller' as they're getting used for other things (the things we are currently doing more often day to day). You're likely wondering why all of a sudden, you've stepped into neuro-speak, but hear me out as this is so important.

Our pleasure is a part of this process and so is our desire. Just like that bicep, we want to strengthen our pleasure pathways by *doing*! And this is where it all ties in.

Remember that bridge we want to build mentioned earlier in part 1? The small-giant steps towards the goal on the other side of the river? The wanting and having sex again? This is how we take that first gigantic and yet seemingly small step.

Focussing on *intimacy* as a way to neurologically 'rewire' our pleasure and wanting is a way to achieve this. Cuddling, kissing, touching, words of love, all of these things I've been discussing throughout this book contribute to your feeling warm, safe and intimate with your partner/lover/yourself and can help reduce the pressure of it all. Plus, it's a way to start creating positive neural associations and remind your brain that you do indeed like and want touch.

I'll be sharing a few really fun, practical ways to do this shortly, but there's a little more explanation I want to give.

Without touch and connection, without affection and feelings of love, warmth and worth, why would we want sex?

Taking a step back, focussing on the little things can remove those psychological barriers to libido discussed earlier, to help you connect, communicate, and maybe then you'll start to feel less 'should-brain' and a bit more 'want-brain'. Differently said, removing the pressure of sex and re-introducing touch, intimacy and affection, is the start of the process that moves sex from something that we *should* do, to something we **want** to do.

Neurologically rewiring our desire, our libido, our pleasure, it takes time and repetition of intimate touch, but it's also extremely simple and enjoyable.

Below I use partner-centric language, but want to confirm that if you're solo and wish to reconnect with yourself and your desire, the below strategies can also be followed with yourself individually, and are also applicable for persons in alternative relationship dynamics.

Where do we start?

Ignore the sex part for now, take it off the table for a timeframe (maybe a month or two), to focus on building that bridge and removing the psychological barriers to wanting. Don't worry, you're only banning sex with each other for a few months, you're welcome to have sex with yourself any time.

I'm sure I sound crazy, 'don't focus on sex to want the sex'. But our brains, our minds, our emotions and psychology are that first step. By removing sex all together from the equation, you're also removing that source of pressure, the 'should-brain', the grief, shame and anxiety. When we agree with a partner that we are temporarily taking sex off the table so we can reconnect, it frees up time for non-agenda'd touch. Touch and affection without the stress of it leading to sex, or going somewhere, allowing you to really enjoy the experience and is powerful for neurological change.

Organise with your lover, partner or yourself time for some touch preferably twice a week following the stages outlined below. This is called 'sensate focus' and is a technique used to reconnect people and increase desire going back to the 60's, created by researchers Masters and Johnson. This process has incredible neurological benefits as it's slow and repeated. The perfect recipe for neurological change.

Stage 1: Start engaging in slow soft touch with each other (or yourself), but clothes on and all over the body. Avoiding typical erogenous zones such as breasts or genitals. But you're taking turns, so one of you is being touched and the other is doing the touch for a limited amount of time (maybe 10 mins each) and then you switch.

Stage 2: Next again is full body slow soft touch, starting with stage 1 touch (avoiding the typical erogenous zone initially).

Then including the erogenous zones over clothing. Still taking turns in touching each other.

Stage 3: This is mutual touching; clothes are optional here. It's important you always start with the type of touch you were doing in stage 1, then 2, then 3 so our body and mind have time to relax and get into it. You're not going for the erogenous zones immediately and you want to avoid orgasms/climaxes and forms of penetration.

Stage 4: If everyone is feeling ready, proceeding through stages 1-3, this 4th stage involves nudity, full body contact and moving into positions that would look like how you would 'normally' have sex (without actually having it). After you've had a few 'sessions' of stage 4 and everyone is comfortable, moving onto having sex (whatever that looks like for you) with each other is fine.

If you keep these touch dates to a few times a week and for 20-40 minutes, you'll start to notice after a few weeks that you're actually looking forward to being touchy and intimate. I've done this myself after treatments to recover my desire and have personally guided others through this process, and it truly does have an effect. It's neuroscience.

The above 4 stages are a guide and depending on which

therapist you see, can vary in what each stage entails and for how long you need to do them. For some the above may sound like something you can try. For others, reading is not doing, and even starting the process to have these conversations or integrate these strategies seems too hard. If that's you, please know I created an online program for couples called 'Connection & Cancer', where I guide and support people through each step of the entire process and more (refer to the 'where to from here' section). Doing is doing, and is where the change really happens, so I've got your back. In the course is a sensate program I designed specifically for people with cancer that spans over six weeks, and doesn't only rebuild desire, but also recovers pleasure sensation and body confidence. Six weeks is the sweet-spot for neurological change as it also allows time to go slow.

If the above doesn't seem achievable for you right now, focus on keeping your intimacy alive. Think of intimacy as the thing that keeps the coals burning, so re-lighting the fire is easier later on. Kiss for the sake of kissing, play the 2-minute game, set a timer and slowly touch parts of each other's bodies. Relearn what you do and don't like. Explore, but also keep it simple. You want to remind your brain that touch and pleasure are things that you can enjoy. This is how we can recreate positive associations to touch and pleasure. We need to remind our brain that we are vessels of pleasure, that we enjoy touch.

Giving ourselves time to understand how our new body works, and the above stages of touch offers slow and effective ways to do that.

There are plenty of affectionate partnerships out there who still struggle with low desire and libido. If this is you, the above sensate therapies are a great way to start that process of wanting again.

A shout-out to partners

Mismatched libido (when one person has a higher libido than the other) is tough. I support partners through so much shame, as they struggle for having desire and libido while their partner is fighting cancer. There is a lot of guilt from this and people quite often do their best to hide their attraction to their partners from this and as mentioned, often looks like distance or disinterest. Libido isn't something that you can switch on and off at will. I know partners who hide when they masturbate from their partner, not wanting to expose them to anything uncomfortable, for feeling like a predator or being interpreted as putting pressure on their loved one. But self-pleasure doesn't have to be solo-pleasure. A partner can pleasure themselves with their loved one lying next to them, or even offering kisses or body touch. This can be beautiful and intimate. This can even influence greater connection and those lusty feelings.

People often simply want to be wanted and loved, and you can show love and affection without it having to lead to sex, which is what so many tools and strategies in this book offer.

Remember, you can have sex without having the sex!

18. CHANGES IN SENSATION

I've been speaking quite generally about how we can rehabilitate our desire and strengthen our pleasure pathways, but I'm going to get a little more specific in this section. In particular, the loss of sensation and erogenous zones through surgeries & treatments, and how losing sensation doesn't necessarily mean losing your sexuality.

I had a breast removed and reconstructed from my lower back tissue nearly two years ago and as I type this, still have no nipple. The breast is firm, a different shape, points in a different direction, feels colder to the touch (could be in my mind) and has zero sensation (not in my mind). Initially, I was in my head about it, feeling self-conscious, embarrassed and anxious (especially the one nipple missing part). Losing breast sensation and pleasure is still hard for me. I miss it; I've lost a piece of my sexuality and I hear this from so many others I support, in reference to not only breasts, but other body parts that have been removed or lost sensation from treatments.

The amazing thing about the human body is that we can create *new* erogenous zones! Remember, our sex and pleasure are what's between our ears and not our legs.

If you're experiencing a loss of sensation due to the removal of a part of your body which would include nerve removal, or your treatments have damaged the nerves, sensation in this particular part of your body may not ever come back. But there is hope.

This is exactly where my bicep theory comes into play. Sensation where nerves are intact is exactly the same as that bicep. You can 'create' new highly pleasurable erogenous zones all over your body, with slow soft touch and being present to how good it feels. Over time, you can have such amazing pleasure from other areas of your body (neck/inner thighs/ears/lips/belly/lower back etc.). How is this done?

Being intimate, focussing on *slow touch* while being curious can start the rewiring process. It's how we create new erogenous zones and enhance pleasure / sensation that may already be there, but just isn't very strong. Play the 2-minute game asking for attention to other parts of your body, offer yourself soft slow touch when you wake up in the morning for 5 minutes each day or if you need extra support, my online course. Your inner thighs can be just as erotic as say, your breasts once were with touch.

I've used the same techniques to help people post-stroke regain sensation on their arms, when working in neurological rehabilitation. With a little repetition and attention, you can enhance your pleasure and sensitivity too. Neurological change doesn't happen overnight, but over time it can and does happen.

Remember, pleasure is still pleasurable, even if it's

somewhere else on your fabulous body.

In the meantime, brain-chatter from things like self-consciousness, anxiety or stress can be the barrier to enjoying touch on your body and also that re-wiring process. If you're getting intimate and feeling self-conscious about your body, pop a little lacy number on, or an item of clothing that's a lovely, sensual material. Something that *feels* nice and helps reduce the anxiety. This will help get your head back into the experience.

Remember, it's okay to get sexy while wearing clothing. Or try some positions that aren't so full-frontal to help you relax and enjoy. The key to enhancing your pleasure, to strengthening those sensory and pleasure pathways is to be present, and we can't do that when we're in our heads.

I also want to note that I have a sense of loss, loss of a part of my body which was a source of *so* much pleasure for me. Please allow yourself time to grieve, process and share how you're feeling. None of this is easy, but the loss of a body part, or loss of sensation on an area of your body doesn't have to mean the loss of your sex or your pleasure all together.

Just like everything else in cancer, it's a process and can take time, but speaking from personal experience as someone who has rehabilitated themselves through these touch practices, it's well worth it.

19. DATING AND CANCER

Dating is scary, I mean even without a cancer diagnosis. And dropping the 'c-bomb' (saying you've had cancer) on a date can get *really* mixed responses like "but you're normal now, right?". It isn't all that bad, there are some people who are incredibly compassionate and respond with kind curiosity, but how do we find them? How do we actually date again without exhausting ourselves while avoiding all the stress and fear?

When it comes to dating, I most certainly am not an expert, so I went and found one. I chatted with dating guru Georgie Wolf, and we came up with some tips.

1: The filter.

Fatigue and low energy levels are a constant after cancer treatments, even years after. The effort of dating apps, the conversations, the actually going on dates only to be disappointed can all be too much. Here's a pro-tip, literally from a dating pro! Say you have or have had cancer *before* the first date. Put things like 'survivor' or whichever words are right for you, on your profile. Mention it in the hello conversation. Additionally, dropping the word 'cancer' may not be the only thing to be nervous about. With varying cancers and their treatments, you may no longer be able to do things like have children or have penetrative sex and knowing when to share these facts can feel daunting. Opening up about these things early on may feel like it will scare some people away (because it will), but this is a good thing because it's a filter. A filter for the people who won't be supportive or understanding, and will waste your time and energy on small talk and dates that go nowhere. You may be reducing the 'pool' so to speak, but a drop in quantity means an *increase in quality*, and this is what we want. Save your precious energy for the actual potentials.

2. Getting naked (or not!).

Our bodies change after cancer, and our confidence and self-esteem can drop. Georgie so insightfully mentions in one of our video discussions, people can have crippling body image issues from other life-events, not just from cancer. If you mention you're nervous, people will respond to that honesty often with understanding, as many of us (most of us) have experienced changes in body image at some point. If they don't respond well to you being open and honest? They're not someone you want to be dating.

One way towards getting more confident about getting naked in front of someone is the first step, the filter. You'll be attracting the type of person who will understand if you say you're a bit nervous to show your body.

Another way to work with your body self-consciousness is

remembering that you don't need to be naked to get intimate. As previously mentioned, you can wear clothes that cover specific body parts (t-shirts, singlets, teddies, sarongs, towels and more). Plus, you can have the lights low and get intimate in positions that aren't full-frontal (which I go into more detail in the sexual positions section in part 3 of this book). This allows you to go slow, not push yourself and reduces that brain-chatter during intimacy. I also discuss strategies to improve self-confidence in detail in the section titled 'body changes & reclaiming confidence' and also a fun way to reduce the fear of undressing in front of others in the upcoming section 'simple ideas for connecting'.

3. Warm-up.

I'm not only talking about foreplay, (which is always necessary and will increase your arousal, desire and sexual confidence with others). I'm also talking about warming-up your **sexual-*self*-confidence**.

- Set yourself a date each week, where you touch your body softly. All over.
- Get a mirror and look at your body, get to know it, but do so with kindness. If you have scars/replaced or removed body parts, look at other parts of your body first...go slow.
- Wear clothing that makes you *feel* good...if you don't have

any, that's okay, buy some.

- Get a few toys that offer pleasure and stimulation to kickstart your sex and sexual confidence (more on that in the toys section in part 3).

- Learning about your body, what it likes and doesn't like is essential for good sex and also, for greater self-confidence and is an important first step to getting your mojo back.

4. Gamify it.

A little bit of structure goes a loooong way, especially with potentially awkward social environments (that's my nice way of saying dates are pretty awkward).

On a date, you could play a question-and-answer game where you take turns asking and answering questions. I love this as a way to get to know people and 'Q&A' (described in the next section) offers a way to 'rig the conversation' to your favour. By that I mean, after a few rounds of the small talk questions covering topics like food and movie interests, ask the question "what's something that's different about your body?". After they've responded and it's your turn to answer, you can describe your body, but do it in a way of amazement. Like, 'how amazing is medicine!' kind of framing. It normalises it, shows that you're okay to talk about it and gives them space to ask questions. This is also brilliant as it starts with your date / the other person telling you something strange about their body first, and you listen with curiosity and compassion. It sets the tone.

If getting naked or showing parts of your body feels scary, do an undressing ritual alone or with a date/lover (detailed in the next section 'simple ideas for connecting'.

If it doesn't go well, you know not to go on another date with them.

5. Baby-stepping towards sex

If you've really hit it off and want to get intimate but are feeling scared, like a broken record I suggest you play the two-minute game (detailed in the next section). I love this game and have been playing it for years including well before, during and after my cancer treatments with partners and also dates. It's brilliant and is the perfect gentle step from enjoying conversation with someone, to enjoying intimacy with someone (without having to leap straight into sex).

These are just a few ideas and suggestions and I truly hope some of the above has been useful to you. It's scary, in so many ways, but there are good people out there.

20. SIMPLE IDEAS FOR CONNECTING

I keep saying connection is possible, but *how* is connection possible? Below I've listed and described some activities that I've taught, read about and love to do - and are my top picks for you to try yourself. It's not an exhaustive list, but will give you a start (i.e., trust yourself and you can decide what works for you). They might not all appeal to you, that is fine. They are varied enough so that hopefully there's something for everyone that seems appropriate to try. And remember, these can be done to the level that is right for you, with the person that is right for you. Some of these can easily be done with a close friend, your carer, by yourself, partners and even family members! It's time to *really* connect. Here's a few ways to do this.

Q&A

I am obsessed with this verbal game and full credit to Roger Butler from Curious Creatures who created it. It's so useful and fun to play if you're in a position where you want to communicate with someone, but it's hard to bring up an awkward topic or start a conversation. It's also great to play any time anywhere, and I love it in social or private settings. It's so simple yet an incredible way to deeply communicate and connect with strangers, loved ones, friends and everyone else.

During many of my treatments, I struggled (and still do) to keep up with conversations that involved more than two people as the brain-fog / cancer-brain had my attention span so low. So, I often played Q&A as a way to be able to listen to one person at a time, and still have valuable, connective conversations with the people around me. Simply put, Q&A makes good conversation great, and when you're struggling, it's a life-saver.

How it works.

Someone asks a question, any question, such as: How was your day? How are you feeling in your body? What do you love about your partner right now? What is your relationship to your sex? Do you like cake more than ice-cream? Anything.

The person sitting to the left of the person who asked the question, answers it first. When they are finished, it goes to the next person to the left, finishing with the person that asked it. There are a few extra rules:

- Every answer is perfect.
- Every question is perfect
- No interrupting someone's answer, wait until they have told you they are finished answering, before sharing your thoughts.
- You can 'pass' on a question (or make something up!).
- You can call 'Tangent' or 'Time' by making a 'T' symbol

with your hands. This indicates that someone may be off on a tangent or taking too much time to answer. We always say "thank you" for a 'T'.

- The person who asks the question, always answers it last.

It may seem strange, having a verbal Q&A game in a book about connection and the importance of intimacy, but there's a theme here. Cancer interrupts life, which includes relationships. Medications, fatigue, nausea, stress, it all interferes and open communication for some can seem too hard. Try this game, try it a few times, it was and still is, a 'go-to' for me, when I want to connect.

Where? You can play it anywhere. Try it in the bath, on the couch, at dinner, in the car or at a BBQ. Play a few rounds at the end of the week to see how you're going. It's a beautiful time to be very honest, because the rules are that you cannot be interrupted and every answer is perfect.

This is also your saving grace if conversations are hard, paying attention is tricky and keeping up with multiple people talking at once. If you let people know what you need and where you're at, they will most likely help you out. I noticed social chatter was a way for people to let me know 'everything was fine'. But it wasn't, I couldn't concentrate, I couldn't follow the conversation, I quickly forgot what people were saying and I got super stressed. As soon as I mentioned I needed conversation to slow down, that's exactly what happened. Remember, you will need to let people know what you need, and they will be grateful for the guidance. Q&A is a brilliant way to have social structure, and still offer wonderful connections with everyone present.

Little, lovely treats

Sit down and write a list of 5 - 10 things that are small and easy to do, that make you feel special or connected to yourself. Little, lovely treats. If you have a close friend or loved one, get them to do the same, write a list of little lovely things they enjoy. This could be a foot massage, a bath, a favourite wine, a nice cheese with salami and a childhood film (my personal favourite), moisturising each other's hands/backs/necks/chests, looking at photos together, a blindfolded touch experience, a game of loving Q&A (just described in this section) or dancing to your favourite music.

So, when a time comes, when you're feeling like you would like to connect, be intimate, share affection and don't know what to do? Get the list out and see what you're in the mood for, or what you're all in the mood for.

All of these small treats should ideally be things that can be done in your home or very close to where you're staying, and don't take a lot of energy. You want your energy to be spent on connecting and enjoying yourself and others' company, not setting up or travelling to a location.

These 'small treats' lists are your go-to. When you're stuck in your head or having a bad day, get the list out. Soak your feet and moisturise them, do yoga, have a self-pleasure session or pleasure a partner, eat an entire pizza when those taste-buds are back online or get your favourite film and a pot of your favourite tea. The point is that you want an easy way to feel special involving yourself, and possibly those close to you. Simple, sensual, special treats that connect you with yourself and possibly others.

Warming and calming

This small yet intimate task can really let you relax, unwind and get connected. A gentle, beautiful way to connect with yourself or with someone else, is by enjoying a warm bath. Relaxing in a body of warm water (not too hot!) has so many positive effects on the body. Muscles relax, our nervous system down-regulates (relaxes), it can reduce stress, muscle tension eases, pain can lessen, blood circulation improves, the list goes on. Add a cup of tea, a glass of wine, something playing on a screen you can see or some quality Q&A (again see earlier in this section) if you have a 'bath-buddy' with you.

The waterless bath

Baths not your thing, or you don't have one? I have for you, the waterless bath experience. Pop your electric blanket on a nice low setting or warm up a heat pack on the couch and create a warm snuggly cocoon for yourself or for you and your pet, child, friend or lover. The intent is to create warmth, intimacy, safety and connection - baths are not essential for this, but feeling safe and snuggly is.

A royal bathing

Credit for this idea goes to my primary carer, who 'softens' the daily activities to connect and show love, and has also used this technique when caring for a friend while undergoing cancer treatments for brain cancer (spoiler, they loved it!). Is your partner, lover, friend or carer helping you with your personal care? Such as dressing, washing or even simply helping you dry your feet after the shower? If this is the case, every once in a while, ask the person assisting with your care to take their time with it. Turn it into an almost worshipping, lovingly sensual dressing or bathing. Imagine the treatment someone might get in a luxury ancient Roman spa.

Slowly wash the feet, slowly caress and wash the back, take your time enjoying putting clothing on someone, let the materials softly brush over the skin. Attention and intention are drivers of pleasure and going slowly allows this to happen. Yes, we are often time poor and we go into 'automatic mode', however this is a lovely five-minute task which can be added into daily life quite easily and shows care, love and affection. This small activity acts as a reminder to each other, you're not in a clinical environment, you're not a nurse going through the rounds with a patient, you're caring for someone, someone you care about. Be soft, be gentle, be present. What a treat and what a connector. And it only needs to take an extra five minutes or so.

A simple good night kiss

Life is hectic and a cancer diagnosis doesn't lighten the load. Finances, appointments, family life, medications, symptoms and more, can fill up the days. The only time you may actually see a partner or lover, is at the end of the day. If this is you, think about taking five minutes, when you're in bed together getting ready for sleep. Lie down facing each other and look into each other's eyes. Touch noses if you like, hold hands, intertwine feet, hold eye contact, share a good-night statement, breathe together or share a kiss on the lips. It's a time where you're both settling down and both in the same spot, it's a great time to use it to connect.

Don't go to bed at the same time as the person you live / share space with? That's okay, ask that you get 'tucked-in' or tuck your partner in. Get the blankets up to their chin, wish them good night, give them a kiss and a few words of love. It's just such a sweet thing. And if you don't share a house with your loved ones? Sweet, loving good night text messages mean the world!

Self-pleasure

Our entire bodies are capable of pleasure and giving yourself some time, some touch and love is a beautiful way to connect with yourself and get those happy chemicals flowing. During treatments you may be tired, stressed, sore, in pain or feeling flat. Whether you're single or partnered, a lovely way to calm and connect with yourself is to give your body, soft, loving touch. This can, but doesn't necessarily need to involve your genitals or you getting aroused. Our bodies are complicated things and treatments can make our body almost feel like a stranger, so getting to know it again can be wonderful.

Give yourself some time, show yourself you're special and set yourself a date. Be it once a fortnight, once a week, or whenever you feel slightly motivated. It's nice, the first few times if you try to leave genitals out of it, just to see what it's like to focus on your body in a different way. We don't give ourselves enough one-on-one time and this is most definitely the case for personal intimate touch. Be curious, explore, hug yourself, scratch, tap, softly touch the skin, find what your body is and is not enjoying, what it does and doesn't enjoy at that moment. I'm a firm believer that offering ourselves self-pleasure, understanding and learning our bodies is essential for us to be able to connect with others. Regardless if you're partnered or not, having some time with yourself is healthy, it's calming, and it's connecting.

Massage swaps

This may seem like a strange thing to recommend in regards to intimacy and pleasure, but hear me out. Touch, care, love and affection are all things many of us forget about during and after treatments. If you're unsure of what your body wants in an arousal, erotic sense, your immediate fallback plan can be massage. Having someone massage you, gives focus on physical, attentive touch without that pressure of it needing to lead to sex. It's pleasurable, it's intimate and gets you connected (and it feels so good!). Massage swaps can also act as an 'ice-breaker', if you're with a partner or on a date and it's been a while since you've touched each other (which is common). This is a lovely and accessible way to ease back into a physical and touch based dynamic without the pressure to 'perform' or 'be sexy'. If you're not partnered and want some touch, but aren't sure how? There are many very skilled professional massage therapists out there, even the 'pop-in' 10-minute massage parlours have amazing touch and anything that connects you to your body and feels good, is a win.

Another amazing benefit of doing massage swaps, is it's a way for a partner or lover to get used to touching your changed body. So often, I support partners through their fear and anxiety of hurting their partner by touching them. A simple massage can be a way to have your partner touch your body and even start to explore areas they are hesitant to touch (like surgery sites or scars). With a little encouragement, direction and permission from you, these fears and anxieties can be overcome, together.

An undressing ritual

Touched on in the Part 2 section 'Body Changes & Reclaiming Confidence', in the top three most common themes I support people through, is changes in body image. How we see ourselves and also, the fear of being naked in front of another person (and ourselves). Undressing rituals are a method of removing clothing for yourself, or another, in a way that is gentle while allowing space for nervousness and shyness and inviting in acceptance and positive regard. You can do this solo by yourself in front of a mirror as a way to get used to your new body, or with a date or partners.

How it works.

There's a lot of scope for variety here so feel free to bend and change this to suit you, but here's the basics. Standing in front of the mirror or someone else, you choose one item of clothing at a time to take off, and as you remove it you make a personal statement. Something that is true, that is how you feel, but also as a way to process, release and move towards acceptance. It's a neat psychological trick and can be wonderful. If you're doing this with a partner, take turns, so after you remove an item of clothing and make a statement, they do the same. Then it's your turn again, and so on.

By statements I mean things like;

- As I remove my shoe, I let go of how hard I am on myself.
- As I take off my shirt, I let go of my self-consciousness.
- Removing my belt is me removing the restrictions of societies ridiculous beauty standards.
- As I remove my bra, I welcome in love and acceptance of my body.
- As I take off my scarf, I release my fear.
- By taking off my pants, I am freeing myself of anxiety.
- By removing my pink sparkly cowboy hat, I am letting go of my tiring day.

Or, if that form of statement doesn't feel right, you could try positive words as you remove clothing and show parts of your body:

- As I look at my arm, I notice the smooth skin I have.

- While looking into the mirror, I'm loving the freckles I have on my face.
- With my chest exposed I feel an appreciation for being alive.
- As I look at my genitals, I notice the awesome curls in my pubic hair.
- As I see my stomach, I see scars/marks of me living, and making it through
- While looking at my lower back, I like the curve where it joins my bottom.

I have done this by myself in front of a mirror, with a long-term partner and also on a date. It was surprisingly effective on the date, as I was very self-conscious about my body and didn't know how to transition from clothed to well, not-clothed. We both took turns slowly removing an item of clothing, we looked into each-other's eyes, we were honest and it was magic. It helped me relax and it helped them understand how I was feeling and how I was struggling.

Go slow. If you're doing this alone in front of the mirror, it can be quite confronting. Don't feel like you need to fully undress, you may need to do this gradually over time. You could remove one additional item of clothing in the mirror to look at and love each time you do this, so it's nice and slow.

I've done it several times alone, as a way to slowly look at myself and get used to my changed and abnormal body. I cried a lot, but it truly helped me with body acceptance and processing my grief for the body I used to have. Follow yourself, breathe and trust that you can stop if you need too. If you're with someone and you don't want to get naked, you can remove 'imaginary' items of clothing (like an orange feather boa, a sequin vest, rainbow suspenders etc.) or simply ask to stop. You could also do this with someone, where you take turns in removing an item of clothing off of the other person, while making positive statements about their body. Or maybe you choose the item of clothing on yourself to remove and your partner/date shares statements of love and appreciation of that particular body part. The best part of this activity, is that there's room to change this to what feels right for you, at the pace that's right for you.

Chatty-massage

If you're liking the ideas in this book about communicating more about what you want and giving more feedback in intimacy and pleasure, but aren't really sure how to do that, this one's for you. 'Chatty massage' is very simple, and is the perfect way to get better at figuring out what you want or don't want, and also, how to ask for it. Plus, this is another excellent activity to do, if your partner is feeling a little hesitant to touch your body, because they're scared of hurting you.

How it works.

Easiest done in pairs, one of you is the 'masseuse', and the other receives the 'massage'. But there's a twist. The person lying down, the one receiving the 'massage' is actually directing the masseuse on what to do. Sounds easy right? Well, there's a little more to it.

The person who is receiving direction, the 'masseuse' is only able to do exactly that, receive and follow directions. They cannot take over the experience or offer what they *think* the person receiving might enjoy. They can only follow the directions given by the person lying down who is 'receiving' the massage. The most important part of this however, is that if the masseuse/person following directions doesn't hear something along the lines of "keep going" or "I like this continue please" or a new instruction, they must stop touching the person giving the directions all together by gently removing their hands and waiting for the next instruction.

Why does the person have to stop touching after 10 seconds of silence you ask? For the person who is receiving the directions, this is a lesson in being guided in touch, in taking feedback and more importantly, not making assumptions as to what the other person may want and 'winging it'. For the person receiving the massage/giving directions, it allows the receiver to learn how to ask for what they'd like and how to communicate if they'd like something to stop, continue or to change. It's powerful stuff. It's also an incredible way for them to really explore their body and to learn what they do and don't like at the pace that's right for them.

Giving feedback and knowing how to receive it during intimacy is the thing that makes a good time, a great time. But we're not taught how to talk about sex or our bodies. We're definitely not taught how to explore our likes and dislikes in a safe and compassionate way. The world would be better if we were. Chatty massage (as simple as it seems) is your way to flex those communication muscles and learn so much about your and your partner's pleasure.

If you're not sure where to start, try doing it together sitting on the couch and just on the hand or shoulders to start with. Or have a clothes-on play together while you get used to how it works. You could even set a timer so you have 5 or 10 minutes each of giving and receiving while you're trying it out. You can start by exploring things like soft touch on your arms, maybe scratchy touch on your back, massage touch on your neck and thighs. Soft kisses on your lower back. Feel free to get creative as the person following directions is going to stop if you don't ask for it to keep going, or for ask for something to change. This is the safety mechanism, so you both can feel free to relax and have a bit of fun with it.

You may be thinking that the more difficult role in this, is the person who's lying down and giving the directions. Funnily enough, when I work with partners together and I teach them this activity it's the complete opposite. It's the person receiving directions and having to stop and withdraw touch after 10 seconds of silence that struggles the most! Due to this, I'm going to repeat the rule as it's surprisingly tough for people, but is so important. If the 'masseuse' doesn't hear a direction after 10 seconds, they must stop what they're doing, remove their hands and wait. This is what will help the person giving direction do exactly that, as they will *have* to give you direction when you stop. So much of our intimacy is guess-work and with the impacts of cancer treatments, clarity and communication has never been more important. Stopping the touch after a short amount of time is a way to help each other practice giving and receiving feedback and most importantly, tuning in to what you do and don't want at the time.

It will 100% feel clunky and awkward at first, just like everything else we try in life for the first time. Don't worry too much about it as this is play, and yes play can be clunky, but it can also be fun. Have a laugh and have another go. Communication is the number one sex move, and this activity is the perfect way to practice.

The two-minute game

Finally, we learn about the two-minute game! I hope how often I've mentioned this game throughout this book gives light to how much I love it. Life coach Harry Faddis created the 'three-minute game' and I was taught the 'two-minute game' from Roger Butler at Curious Creatures, and it's simply brilliant. This game is suitable for those experiencing treatment and their loved ones, is great when you have no idea how to connect with someone or where to start and is a wonderful way to gently get to know each other's bodies again.

Here's the rules.

- Set a timer or an alarm on your phone for two minutes.
- Pick who goes first, then that person asks for something they would like for 2 minutes (some examples are listed shortly).
- If you all agree, start the timer and give the person whatever they asked for.
- When the timer goes off, completely stop what you're doing.
- Then it's the next person's turn to ask for something they would like for two minutes.
- If everyone agrees, start the timer and go.
- Once the timer goes off, again, stop what you're doing.
- And repeat.

That's it. Really, that is the game. So simple, yet so effective. You can play it for as long as you like - 10 minutes or an hour, or however long you have energy and are having fun. Time can really fly when playing this game.

Also, this game can be played with anyone, not just someone you're in a relationship with. It could be a friend, family member, carer and doesn't have to be in pairs. There are so many ways to connect, to touch and be touched, which this game can help you discover.

One of the first (out of possibly hundreds) times I played this, I wasn't sure what to ask for. So, of course, I asked for a shoulder massage. Then, that became a slow back scratch. Then full body soft touch and I was amazed at how starting simply and being left wanting more (thanks to that timer) guided me to what I would like next. Asking for what you want can be difficult at first, but this game allows you to develop that skill with practice and repetition, and asking for what we want is such an essential skill to have during cancer treatments (and always).

A common question when introducing the two-minute game in workshops is, "what happens if someone asks for something you don't want to do?" Say "no-thank you" with a smile and discuss an alternative (such as touching the chest or back rather than genitals). It's okay. Wait, it's more than okay, it's wonderful to say 'no'. Saying what we don't want is equally (maybe more) important than saying what we do want. The goal is to find that optimal place where everyone is happy giving and receiving.

Here's a few reasons why this game can work for you:

Our genitals aren't always up for being played with, so when it's your two minutes, ask for something that doesn't include them (you have your whole body).

This game can allow connection, even with different levels of libido. Someone might want sexual touch for two minutes and if you're happy to give it, great! Your two minutes could be something that suits your mood such as 'tell me your favourite joke using your hand as a puppet'. The possibilities are endless and you can ask for exactly what you want, while avoiding what you don't want.

Bodies impacted by treatment can change dramatically and unpredictably, be it sensation, arousal, pain, surgical sites etc. This game allows you to relearn how your body works or doesn't work (where those desensitised parts are, where it's sore, where it's pleasurable, how toys or lubes feel).

If you're playing this with a partner and are worried about where things may lead to? Take 'typical' sex off the table for the entire game. You could have a 'no genital contact' rule or even leave your clothes on. Remove the pressure to perform or get aroused. Obligation & expectation are the enemy of arousal, feeling safe and relaxed is its catalyst. Get creative, enjoy yourselves without that pressure. You can enjoy pleasure from soft intimate touch anywhere on the body.

The two-minute game has many communication benefits and can act as a gentle ice breaker. With changed sexuality and changed intimacy (with or without illness), can come distance and avoidance. Talking about sex is not easy, especially when things are different. This game gently offers a way to help navigate those tricky feelings while also acknowledging the elephant in the room. While we're at it, let's erase any feelings of 'being selfish' or 'a taker'. Asking for your neck to be gently kissed for two minutes, or to be told why this person loves you for two minutes, is simply playing the game. It can seem difficult, but remember, you have to ask, it's the rules! Through my work as a sexuality and consent workshop facilitator, I'm always shocked at how many people tell me that they have never asked for what they want before. Practice makes perfect and it does get easier the more you do it.

Here's a list of things you could ask for, for your two minutes:

- Can you please lower the lights, put some relaxing music on that I would like, bring me water and join me on the couch in two minutes?
- Hold my hand and tell me how you're doing for two

minutes.

- Massage my (insert body part here) for two minutes.
- Starting at my neck, ever so softly touch my entire body, back to feet over two minutes.
- Tell me about your day through interpretive dance.
- Put on a song and show me your silliest/favourite dance move.
- Make me a cup of tea in two minutes.
- I would like to cuddle for two minutes.
- I would like to offer you a shoulder massage for two minutes (that's still your two minutes, but if you're not up for being touched, you can touch others. It's all about what YOU want)
- Massage my head.
- I would like to stroke your hair with your head in my lap.
- Lightly touch my beautiful bald head for 2 minutes.
- Gently kiss my neck/chest/thighs/back for two minutes.
- Show me how you like to be kissed, for two minutes.
- Kiss my face and tell me things you love about me for two minutes.
- Softly breathe on my entire body, ending with my genitals for two minutes (YUM!).

If you're thinking, "ugh, whatever Tess. Some of us

don't know how to just simply know what you want and ask for it." You're right, I hear you. None of us are taught this, but I have a solution for you. A beautiful baby-step towards the 2-minute game and flexing those 'asking' muscles, is by playing the previous activity 'chatty massage'.

Active receiving

'Active receiving' is a way to connect with a lover/partner to the level that is right for you, when you're not feeling sexy or like having sex and maybe need a little bit more time to get those feelings flowing.

It's a one-way touch experience, and a great way to enjoy touch, especially if you're not feeling 'sexy'. I'll explain a little more. There are many expectations and misconceptions in intimate activities, and a super common one is that it should always be a two-way experience. You give and receive pleasure at the same time. Well, this doesn't necessarily always have to be the case, and I offer you a wonderful way to connect in a one-way touch format, very similar to 'chatty massage' mentioned previously. This is wonderful for people with mismatched libido, delayed arousal responses (detailed in the 'reactive versus proactive arousal' section in Part 3), if someone is not wanting to receive intimate touch or may not know what they want at that moment, but would love to see a partner have pleasure and enjoy themselves.

How it works.

Someone lies/sits down (or is in any comfortable position), asks for what type of touch they want, and constantly directs that person in how they touch them. The other person does exactly what they are being told to do. That's it! It's incredibly fun and accessible.

Imagine the person giving the touch and receiving the directions has no mind of their own, they are an inanimate object that only responds to commands. For the person following instructions, it can free you from that common brain chatter ("am I doing this right? Are they enjoying this? Are they pretending?"), as you're just doing what you're told.

Some examples of directions the person who is receiving touch (and giving all directions) could give are: "Massage my shoulders. Can you now scratch my back? Yum, thanks, can you go slower and a bit firmer? Softly touch my body up and down, neck to feet with your fingertips and don't stop until I say. Now, lightly pinch my inner thighs. Breathe cool breath on my nipples." Anything you want, just ask.

Unlike in chatty massage where the person following directions stops all together if they don't hear anything after a short while, the person giving the touch can check in to see if it's how they want it ("How is this pressure? Would you like me to move my hands, faster or slower?"). The person following directions doesn't change anything, doesn't alter any style without being directed. If the person giving touch doesn't receive any directions for a while and isn't sure if this is still what the person receiving still wants? Keep doing what you were last asked to do and ask the question "how could you enjoy this more?".

Similar to chatty massage, this is an incredible skill to learn in the bedroom. Giving directions, asking for what we want, checking in with a lover to get feedback on their level of enjoyment, communicating your desires, all of this leads to better communication and better sex. If you get tired? Simply stop the activity whenever one of you wants. The goal is to enjoy receiving and to enjoy giving. 1 minute, 10 minutes, 20 minutes, it's all perfect.

If you're unsure, give it a go, clothes on, on the couch, using just an arm or hand. Practice following directions, practice giving directions, practice checking in and identifying what you want. There is no goal here, just to have a touch experience, to give or receive pleasure, and enjoy connecting with a partner. It may feel clunky at first, but with practice it flows very easily and you will be amazed at how much you learn about your partner and their body (and yours!).

If this sounds like fun to you, but asking for what you want and giving directions seems a bit daunting, or taking directions and not being the one driving the experience sounds tough, I recommend playing 'chatty massage' or the '2-minute game' a few times first, before jumping into this activity. I say this only because it won't be enjoyable if you're still getting used to these styles of intimate communicating. Those two activities are a wonderful (and fun!) way to develop these amazing sexy skills.

21. WHAT HAVE WE COVERED?

- The knowledge for loved ones that we won't break if you go in for a hug and how to communicate that.

- Navigating body-image changes, fatigue, pain, understanding the impacts treatments such as chemotherapy, radiotherapy & hormone treatments can have.

- How things like sensation, pleasure and desire can be recovered.

- Dating and strategies to reduce the stress and effort for your successes.

- Specific examples of how you can connect with others, including activities with just yourself or with others, ranging from purely verbal exercises to ones including touch.

PART 3: LET'S GET SEXY

This section takes a look more directly at sex. I address, not only topics such as communication, vaginal atrophy, changes in erection and some sex-myth busting, but I also look at physical positioning to get around some tricky symptoms.

Not only have I fought cancer myself, but being an OT trained in sexuality and sexology, I really have walked my talk. I've learnt so much through 'being my own patient' so to speak, and am delighted to share these approaches and solutions with you.

What I cover in this section:

- Some of the impacts I suffered and conquered.
- Communicating about sex.
- Letting go of sexual shame and taking sex less seriously.
- Fairy sex-tales (myths and misconceptions).
- Delayed arousal responses.
- Changes and loss of orgasm.
- Vaginal atrophy and pain.
- Changes in erection.
- The varied types of lubes, including which one's best when.
- Some information on hygiene and personal care.
- Sexual positioning, techniques and tools.
- And toys!

After reading Part 3, you will have communication tools to discuss sex, physical positioning ideas so you can engage in sex even with all of those side effects, and even information about safer sex and how to bring it up with your treating team. Don't let your sexual side fall silent and go into hibernation. Part 3 of this book is where what you thought was sexually impossible, becomes possible.

22. HOW TREATMENTS AFFECT YOUR SEX LIFE

I thought I'd share a little about my experiences during treatments, to give a little context as to how sexuality can be affected.

Chemotherapy gave me labia ulcers and vaginal pain which made even a fingertip of penetration cause unbearable pain. Hemorrhoids prevented anal play and nausea had me wanting to keep still while constantly sipping on frozen cokes for instant relief. Mouth ulcers and bleeding gums had tasks such as eating challenging, so kissing was definitely not on the table. Endocrine treatments gave me vulva and vaginal atrophy so bad, there were days and weeks I was unable to walk, sit-down, or wear underwear or pants (I haven't ridden my bicycle in years). I also have joint and bone pain and regular migraines. Chronic pain from radiotherapy and fatigue, drain tubes, surgery sites, and so much more. As you can imagine during these times, sexual activities were not something I was craving. However, with the guidance in this part of the book, you will find some solutions.

It's important to note that it's not just treatments which can lower our libido, cause changes in arousal and orgasm, but also medications. It's okay, you may still be able to enjoy a lot of pleasure, maybe even have orgasms (just different ones) in ways that might surprise you. Also, this is an important time to remember, you can still have pleasure and arousal without having to reach climax. Again, I repeat, pleasure is pleasurable!

One of the most common lessons I teach and other sexuality therapists teach, is that sex is more than your genitals, sex is more than your orgasm. Sex is your body, your connection, your arousal, your pleasure, your touch, your giving and your receiving.

23. COMMUNICATING ABOUT SEX

I've mentioned that you will need to be your own sexual advocate and have given many samples for how to ask questions, but it really is so important you do ask them. I'm not just referring to your treating team, but with those around you that you're intimate with. It can seem daunting, which is why I've been littering this book with specific communication examples. In part 3, I also include a wonderful, fun activity you can do with a partner or lover, even if you're not up for the 'typical' form of 'sex'. More on that soon.

Why you should ask your health care team?

I'm continually asking you to speak up to your treating team, because if you wait for someone to bring it up, it may not happen. Through an almost complete lack of healthcare professionals initiating a conversation on this topic, I learned that I needed to take the initiative myself to ask the questions. Given how important the topic of intimacy, relationships, sexuality and well-being is, don't be shy - always ask, and if you need to, persist. Medical staff may not voluntarily bring it up, but I've found they are often very well-informed once I ask and are more than happy to have those conversations.

I once asked a nurse while I was in the chemo-chair for advice regarding the ulcers I had on my outer labia. The response I got was calm and not shaming at all, she said she would "ask around" and walked off. She didn't return for over half an hour, so of course I thought she might have been embarrassed and was avoiding the topic, and due to that, I was reluctant to bring it up again. When she eventually returned and didn't mention it, I plucked up some courage and asked her again. The nurse apologised immediately and explained that there was a medical emergency in the next room and it had slipped her mind. She went out to ask the person she was originally going to ask, came back quickly with information, I wrote down the recommendation for a topical cream and everything was fine.

I'm so glad I persisted because my assumption was wrong. The nurse was perfectly happy to discuss it with me, she was just preoccupied with something else. This is a perfect example of how you will need to advocate for yourself and for information about sexuality in clinical settings. Sometimes it's not a priority, but most of the time the staff are so very busy, working tirelessly and these things take a backseat. Another thing that was a pleasant surprise was that the nurses, surgeons, radiologists and pharmacists I spoke to didn't blink an eye when I asked them sexuality-based questions. And they were more than happy to contact the relevant medical professional to answer any questions when they weren't sure what recommendations to give. Medical professionals are trained to talk about bodies, bodily functions and intimate things as part of their job, so, be confident that all you need is to pluck up the courage to ask.

If you do come across a health professional who is uncomfortable when you ask a question or bring up the topic, my suggestion is not to take this personally and just ask someone else, or ask that person who else you could speak with. We've all been brought up with shame around sex and for some healthcare professionals, despite their values and training, might still feel embarrassed. This doesn't have anything to do with you, so please don't take it as a reason to not ask others. You'll find the people around you who are particularly helpful and forthcoming with assistance, I recommend writing their name down so you can focus on directing any questions to them.

Communicating with your partners

Pop-quiz, what am I?

We're not supposed to talk about it, you can't have too much of it, you can't have too little of it, it's used in nearly all marketing to sell but it's never presented accurately in the media, it's a part of human life, social media platforms shut you down for talking about it, people who are different, unwell, older, living with disability, are of different cultures and ethnicities are assumed to not have it or to want it, we receive no education on it yet we're supposed to magically be good at it and we're supposed to always want it……. Yup. That'd be sex.

You may feel from reading the above that you can't win, and sure, our culture doesn't exactly embrace open communication regarding sexuality, but reading this book is how you will learn.

In my experience as a sexuality educator (as well as from my own life), people who are able to talk between themselves about sex more openly, have much better sex. Why, you ask? Because communicating about how you're feeling and what you might enjoy, allows you to engage comfortably and pleasurably. It can also reduce feeling like you're forcing yourself, forcing someone else, or causing any possible harm. It's okay if things have changed, our bodies and pleasure always will. If we can learn how to communicate about what we do or don't want, things will be better. Remember, hand holding, eye contact, cuddles, snuggles on the couch, foot/body/hand massage, genital massage, oral genital play, assisting/giving masturbation, self-touch together, watching pornography together or reading erotic literature together, all of these things are sex and all of them are connective.

I'm going to share a story of someone who wrote about their experience of sex after having their penis removed due to cancer. Post-surgery, he and his wife still have regular sex and are even more satisfied with the quality of their intimacy than before. He shared that before cancer he would ejaculate every time they had sex, which would last around 15 minutes. Now, he has orgasms from his nipples, thighs and scrotum being touched (how amazing is the neuroplasticity of pleasure!). He also now offers his wife many more orgasms and their sex lasts on average an hour. He refers to it as more "quality". They communicate more, explore each other's bodies more and pleasure each other more. A changed body doesn't necessarily mean worse sex or the end of it all together, change can have its rewards.

24. LET'S TAKE SEX LESS SERIOUSLY!

You might think that things like fatigue or nausea are the number one thing to get in the way of us being sexual during treatments. But as I've touched on previously, it's also shame, embarrassment, that 'should-brain' and naming that elephant in the room.

The most important lesson in this book

Here's a step towards breaking the silence and awkwardness around openly talking about something we've been raised to think should be a subject only for private hushed ears.

Sex at times (most of the time) is clumsy and it's messy. We humans cannot read minds and with sex being complex enough, when you add cancer treatments into the mix? Communication is never more important. We are raised to think that sex should be a secret, something to be embarrassed or awkward about. Well, those times are over. To get through your treatments and maintain connection, a dialogue needs to happen. Talking about your sexuality and your intimacy *must* happen. This goes for someone during and after treatments, or a partner, carer or lover of someone going through treatment. Communication is key.

So, on that note, I have a favour to ask you. No, scrap that. There's something you must do, before you continue reading.

If you're in a private location, alone or with someone you trust, I want you to say the word 'sex' out loud 10 times (maybe don't do this while you're in the taxi or the hospital waiting room). But wait! Each time you say it, I want you to say it while pulling silly faces and using different voices. High pitches, low pitches, squeaky voices, growling the word, howling the word, but no matter what, you cannot say the word 'sex' and try to be sexy.

If you're alone, do it in the mirror. If you have a friend, sibling, parent, partner or lover in the room, look up and say to them "Tess says we need to say the word 'sex' at each other in stupid voices, pulling stupid faces 10 times each". They of course will immediately stop what they're doing (because I said so!), and complete this task with you.

So, let it out and let it out weird!

Have you done it? (I hope the answer is yes).

Now, I want you to look around. You just said the word 'sex' out loud, maybe with someone else in the room, and have you noticed that the roof did not collapse? The world has not caught on fire and the Universe continues on?

I asked you to do this for a few important reasons. As mentioned above, addressing sexuality, sexual challenges and intimacy concerns requires communication, whether with an intimate partner or a medical professional. And how can we communicate about sex if we have trouble saying the word? Well, now you know, that's all it is. It's just another word. You've said it, 10 times out loud in a weird and bizarre way and the world didn't explode. Plus, saying 'sex' while pulling faces and making silly voices is a very important reminder to you. A reminder that, just like this activity, sex can be awkward, clunky, hilarious, creative, done alone, done with others, you don't have to be 'sexy' to engage in sex and…it can be fun.

Well-done!

Sexual Shame

As touched on in part 1, shame is a pretty useless emotion, but can run rampant during life's tougher moments. There are so many ways shame can pop up and be that never ending nagging weight in our minds. I now want to give voice to the other elephant in the room known as 'sexual shame'.

Sexual shame commonly stems from those feelings that we are not good enough or that we are flawed in some way. Guess what? We *are* flawed. We are human, and you (carer, lover, patient) are going through a very, very unpredictable and challenging time. For people with partners during cancer treatments, mismatched libido's/sexual drive can be quite common. So, I'm just going to say it. You're not a bad person for wanting sex, you're not a bad person for not-wanting sex. You're not a bad person for not wanting to talk about something that is causing discomfort and negative emotions. You're not a bad person for struggling.

I was very ashamed at times. I put a lot of pressure on myself to 'do better' as I felt like I *'should* do better'. I'm a sexuality educator and clinician for crying out loud, I *should* want sex during all my treatments, right? Wrong. It was hard to come to terms with this, I felt flawed for struggling, I felt flawed for my decreased libido, I felt flawed for what I perceived as 'letting people down' by not being connected or engaged with people during treatment. During treatments, my sexual desires decreased and thoughts such as 'what's wrong with me?' increased. Wow, isn't it amazing, how hard we can be on ourselves?

When we're in partnerships with others and there are different levels of desire, there can be many, many different forms of shame. These will look pretty familiar from the examples of psychological barriers to libido discussed in part 1 however want to repeat these as it's pretty important.

There's often shame associated with:
- wanting sex
- not wanting sex

- saying no
- saying yes
- making offers of sex and possibly worrying that you're harassing your unwell partner
- body shame, and not wanting to be intimate with others
- changed arousal
- changed libido
- putting your needs before someone else's.
- needing so much self-care

Other causes of shame:

- not wanting to be hugged
- not wanting to see friends
- telling someone you don't want them to come over because you're too tired
- being unwell
- needing help
- asking for help
- not asking for help
- not being able to communicate with the people around you
- not doing 'better'
- shame for having shame!

If you're experiencing sexual changes and feeling shame, remember this. Never, ever force yourself to engage sexually to overcome guilt, shame or to do someone a 'favour'. It won't be enjoyable for you, or the other person. You're (all) likely to have a negative experience and afterwards, may be at risk of more unpleasant emotions like regret. Plus, remember, if we force ourselves to have sex and don't enjoy it, our brain will start to neurologically rewire and associate sex as a negative experience and you will *want it less.*

Find a professional, a support person, or a loved one to share with. Don't keep things bottled up or they will explode, and can in time show themselves in other ways, such as anger, hatred, temper tantrums or ultimatums. None of which will improve the situation, or bring you closer to those around you. It's so important to speak with someone. Ask your doctor or oncologist if the hospital has a psychologist or counsellor you can see. If they don't? Ask to see the hospital social worker and discuss a referral to see someone in the community. Supports are essential and they are out there, ask your treating team to help you find them.

Another form of sexual shame, may be for those who have penises and are experiencing changes in function. Our culture has told many of us that a hard penis means enjoyment, an erect penis means that things are 'going well'. Soft penises to some are regarded as non-sexual, that a person needs to 'try harder to get hard' or a soft-cock means that they don't find you attractive or don't want to be intimate with you. A soft or hard penis is hard to hide, you're exposed and so is your 'arousal'. I feel for you, and I'm so truly sorry if you have ever experienced shame due to your delightful, sensual, soft-penis.

News flash everyone: a soft penis is delicious, sensitive and can still experience pleasure. As the giver of sexual touch to a soft penis, it can be (and is) extremely pleasurable to offer pleasure and play, without things needing to be hard or erect. Plus, it's also very enjoyable for the receiver. You can orgasm without an erection and you can orgasm without a prostate gland if you don't have one. I say this as someone who coaches people post prostatectomy (prostate removal) on exactly this. How to experience pleasure and orgasm with a soft-penis and rehabilitate function (refer to the resources section and 'A Touchy Subject' for more on that).

To anyone that has seen a soft penis and said out loud or thought in their head "what's wrong?", please, please, don't think this way. The pressure of getting erect can be the thing that interferes with the process of getting erect. After surgeries, medications, chemo, stress, fatigue & pain, getting erect may be difficult. Please understand, soft-penises are wonderful, sexy and still capable of pleasure.

Of course, if there are ongoing issues, consult your doctor, but being hard doesn't mean you're 'good' at sex, for the giver or for the receiver. Being good at sex isn't about how hard you get, or how hard you make someone else get, it's about how you touch, communicate, offer and enjoy pleasure.

25. FAIRY SEX-TALES

Before we go any further, I thought I'd address some common misconceptions around sex and intimacy, which can get in the way of our pleasure. I see these misconceptions all the time with clients and I've seen people's sex lives transform by realising there's more to what we have often been led to believe when it comes to 'sex'. If you already know these, then yay! If some or all of them are new to you, then yay for learning new ideas!

Having sex with someone could give them my cancer

The good news here is that cancer is not a sexually transmitted infection or disease. You can't give it to the person you're intimate with. We must always act safely in sex, as there are other things which are transmissible, but your cancer is not one of them.

A partner/lover should know what I want, or, I shouldn't have to ask

Humans are not mind readers and our own wants, moods, desires and ways we feel can, and do, change. They can change over time, even from moment to moment. We tend to learn what our partners like and dislike better over time but you can't expect anyone to magically know what you want at any given moment. This is even more the case when something causes changes in our bodies, such as treatments. It's important to communicate with our partners: to tell each other what we want and to ask our partners/lovers what they want or might enjoy.

Sex must end in orgasm

A myth about orgasms is that you must have one for sex to be good. Sure, orgasms are great but they are not essential and the presence of an orgasm doesn't mean you're 'good at sex' (whatever that means). One of the most common things impacting people's ability to orgasm is not genital size or shape. It's not technique either. It's our state of mind. Pressure, obligation and expectation gets in the way of our arousal, it doesn't encourage it. As previously mentioned, when we let go of the need to orgasm, when we free our minds of that agenda, that can often be the thing that allows them to happen.

Only people with a penis ejaculate

It doesn't matter what shape your genitals have, we all have the potential to ejaculate (come) and yes, vagina's can squirt. Direct stimulation on the internal erogenous zones (like the g/a/pspots) and for some, cervix or clitoral, can influence ejaculation. We're all unique in our pleasure.

Squirting, orgasm, ejaculation, it's all the same

If you have a penis, a vulva, or anything and everything in between, orgasms and ejaculation don't have to go hand in hand. They can, and do, happen separately for some. For those with a penis, this is not necessarily a skill you're born with, but with training and practicing control, this is a skill most can learn. Vagina's squirt is not urine, can be clear or cloudy in presentation, and range from a dribble to a projectile. No matter what your genital configuration, orgasms and ejaculating can be together and/or separate.

If your genitals aren't working as usual then you can't orgasm

Firstly, orgasms occur in the brain. Secondly, there's more than one type. People have orgasms from stimulation on the scrotum, the anus, the penis, clitoris, vagina, G-spot (urethral sponge), a-spot, p-spot, prostate gland, cervix, a-typical forms of genitalia, nipple play, from breath, neck touch, foot touch, ear nibbles, inner thighs…the list goes on. I've even seen someone have a full body orgasm, from laughing in their pleasure and no physical contact whatsoever. A laugh-gasm! If cancer treatments are hampering you from orgasming like you used to, the good thing is that bodies can orgasm in lots of different ways. It just might take some patience while you try new things.

The G-spot guarantees orgasm

The G-spot is not an anatomical structure, but is part of a larger internal network of structures. This term refers to an internal zone where some (not all) experience pleasure when it's stimulated. Roughly a finger nail / first knuckle depth inside the vaginal canal, up top / the stomach side of the body (anterior). It feels like the rough tissue just behind your top teeth. Pushing on this 'area' doesn't guarantee an orgasm. For those that do experience pleasure in this area, it requires warm up, blood-flow to the area and time to get aroused (like everything else with pleasure). It's not an 'on switch', it's a *possible* erogenous zone or pleasure point. The surrounding areas also need to be stimulated and aroused for this area to become sensitive (which makes sense, as it's said to stimulate our internal clitoral-body structures). Once the internal tissues and structures are aroused and have engorged from blood-flow, some people can have orgasms and even perhaps ejaculate. For others, this particular area doesn't trigger orgasmic experiences at all. If you don't experience 'G-spot' pleasure, you're normal as many don't. Like everyone, we have pleasure points all over our bodies and everyone is different.

There are other internal erogenous zones such as the a-spot which is the same side of the vaginal canal as the G-spot, but further in and the p-spot, inside the vaginal canal pointing in the direction of the anus. For people with prostates, the p-spot is easily accessed inside the rectum about your first finger knuckle in or a tad more in the direction towards the abdomen (feels like a walnut). These are all names for areas that for some (not all) can be highly pleasurable.

Anal sex hurts and isn't pleasurable

This was heartbreaking to type, but I've heard this perspective often. Your anus has the potential for so much pleasure! Here's the deal, anal sex will hurt if it's not done well, just like other forms of sex. The anus needs love and attention, and wow can it feel great. Like anything in sex, warm up is vital and for anything anal, lubricants are *essential*. If we go slow, take our time and let our body relax into touch and sensation, pleasure can come. If you feel pain, stop. Remember? "No pain, *no pain*". There are minimal risks to having an 'accident' when you're playing with this area, however if you're nervous, wear gloves, get a towel underneath you, engage after a bowel movement or you can even give yourself an anal douche. These options aren't vital, but may help calm your mind if you're worried. A way to safely start exploring your anus is in the shower or bath, giving yourself a soft massage. Gently massage all around the anus, the butt cheeks, softly stretch the anus and lightly touch it, go slow. Anal pleasure is for everyone, be curious and explore, you may be very, very surprised. A client and I explored alternative forms of pleasure as the anti-depressants she was on were blocking her clitoral & vaginal orgasms. What she learnt was by resting the tip of an extra-small vibrating butt plug against her anal entrance (not even going inside), she was able to experience intense pleasure and even orgasm.

If you have had bowel or pelvic surgeries, it is vital you ask your surgeons the recommended time you should avoid anal-play, so you can heal.

Self-pleasure is pointless, I need a partner to have sex

Self-pleasure is essential and you don't need to have a partner to have sex. Even if you do have a partner, many sex therapists will still recommend you self-pleasure anyway. Why? Giving yourself time, touch and connection is a way for you to relearn your body and also enhance pleasure. Just like when we stop practicing a language we are learning and over time we forget it, it's the same with our pleasure. Treatments or no treatments, we need to continually engage with ourselves, connect with ourselves, our sensations and our pleasure so we don't *lose it*. With more practice, with more knowledge of your body, desire can also increase. Regular self-pleasuring is a very useful tool when wanting to recover from changed sexual drive and changes in pleasure.

If I need sexual services, it's wrong to pay for them

It's okay to pay for the services you need. Humans need love and affection and during cancer treatments, isolation and loneliness can occur. There can be times when we need companionship and connection and it's just not available to you. If you're solo, independent, or your relationship agreements support external intimacies, seeing a sex-worker can be clean, simple and safe. A transactional experience, where you can ask for what you want, get it, and then head home. Simple and satisfying. Sex-workers offer affection, cuddles, touch, and yes, also sex, which are all things you have a human right to access. Plus, sex-workers often have a lot of experience working with body limitations. If this world is of interest but seems scary, I highly recommend looking at this resource 'satisfactionproject.com'.

26. REACTIVE AROUSAL VERSUS PROACTIVE AROUSAL

I've discussed in part 2 mismatched libido, but I'd also like to discuss mismatched arousal. Remember, arousal is the way our body responds *in* pleasure. As mentioned in part 1, arousal responses could include things like an increase in heart rate, our pupils dilate, skin sensitivity increases, tissues become engorged, we become wet, we become hard and more.

Delayed arousal responses are extremely common from treatments and medications, and can also be caused by many psychological aspects like stress and nervousness. Just like we have the many layers (physiological, psychological and neurological) that can impact our libido, so do these layers potentially impact our arousal. What this can look like, is you don't 'want it as much' (or at all), it takes a lot longer for you to 'get into it' than it used to. That you notice it feels like maybe you're forcing yourself at the start, but after some time, things start to feel more enjoyable. Sound familiar?

I call this '**reactive** vs **proactive**' pleasure and arousal.

Reactive means, in *response* to something. You *react* to a thing or stimulus. With arousal and pleasure, that could look like only feeling aroused *after* you have been kissing and touching for some time. You're reacting to the touch and intimacy.

Proactive means something that happens *without* prompt or stimulus. It happens without needing something to react too. In pleasure and arousal this could look like you're watching television and all of a sudden, you're gagging for it. Or you walk down the street enjoying the sun on your face and you then notice your underwear is damp and the breeze feels soooo good!

Countless people feel their enjoyment of sex is gone forever, that they have lost their desire completely because their pleasure and arousal seem now absent (is no longer proactive). But in actual fact, it's just now reactive and it needs something to respond to and a bit of time to kick in. There's a gigantic difference between someone who doesn't enjoy sex at all versus someone who needs time to enjoy it.

I support many who think they cannot stand sex at all anymore and are desperate to reclaim this part of their life, and when I ask "So what do you do to warm-up before sex," this question is followed by silence, a tumbleweed rolls past and that's the moment where I get my whiteboard out.

I'd like you (and anyone you're with) to grab a piece of paper and a pen, a notebook, or anything you can individually draw and write on. Now, draw a very basic XY graph (just a small graph is fine) with the Y axis labelled as 'arousal' and the X axis labelled as 'time'.

It should look something like this:

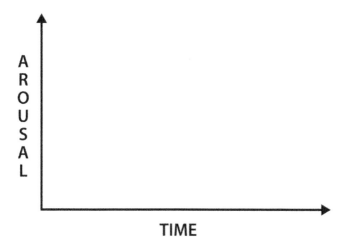

This graph is going to represent how much time we need for our arousal and pleasure to kick-in, once we've started touching and playing either with ourselves or a partner. We're tracking our arousal response. As you move to the right, this indicates time passing. As you move upwards, this indicates your level of arousal increasing.

Imagine now, that you're getting sexy with yourself or a partner. This is where we're at the very start of the graph, where X & Y connect at the bottom left. I want you to draw a line on this graph, starting at this point, that shows what you feel your current arousal response is over time. You could get specific with this if you like, but mostly, let's just use this broadly as a guide and note that this graph could represent around an hour of time.

To repeat the task, imagine you're getting intimate with yourself or a partner. I want you to draw on the graph, a line representing what you think your arousal and pleasure response is like over time.

Here's an example of what this *could* look like:

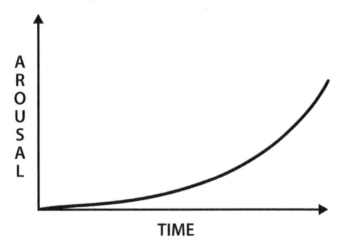

This graph shows that this person doesn't have an immediate arousal response (which is very normal during and after treatments), however after some time and a bit of lovin, they start to enjoy things more.

Now, if you're currently doing this with another person, I'd like for you to draw a second graph, and on this one, you're going to redraw your own line on it, and also in the same graph in another colour, copy this other person's line into it also. Then, circle where those lines intersect (if they do). So, you have two (or maybe more if you're with multiple people) lines on the one graph, giving us a comparison.

It *could* look something like this:

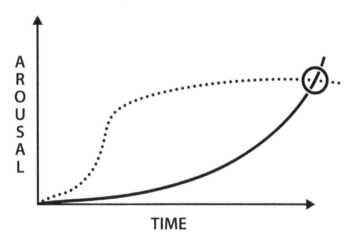

For many people the lines vary quite a bit and for others, not so much. There's no right or wrong here, we're simply visualising the invisible processes within our body. No matter how similar or different these lines are, it's extremely rare that the lines would be identical.

Why? Because we are all different, as is our sex and our

pleasure. But the two parts of this graph I want you to focus on is the part where the lines intersect, and the space in between the lines which I've highlighted.

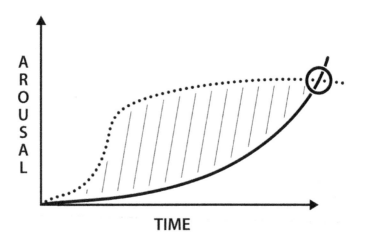

The space in between the lines represents the time in your connection and intimacy, where you're mismatched in your pleasure and arousal. One of you is more aroused, faster. What we want to do is get you to the point where those lines intersect, because this is your happy spot. This is where sex is pleasurable and enjoyable for all involved. This is the sexy goldilocks zone.

That highlighted space is the guide for you to know how much more time and attention one person needs, so you can get to that intersection point for mutual enjoyment. This is fantastic to know, because guess what? If you need more time and attention, we can give you more time and attention!

Brainstorm together, right now, some things you can do together or alone, that will help the person who needs a little more time, to feel relaxed, feel calm and feel sexy. What things could you do at the start of your play and intimacy that will help this person arrive into their body and pleasure, so you're both on the same page? Is it a massage? A warm bath followed by some soft touch? Is it soft kisses on the neck and lower back? Is it watching some porn together? Use that space in the graph, the mismatch in your pleasure as a guide on how to get your pleasure to match. This is how sex becomes more enjoyable for everyone and ties into the thing that will contribute you to wanting it more. Remember that bicep? The wanting? If we're having lovely experiences with ourselves/partners, we will be creating those positive pleasure neurological associations and want it more!

For people doing this individually, look at the curvature of your line/arousal. Is there a lot of time where you aren't feeling pleasure and those arousal responses? Think about your self-pleasure practices. Are they rushed? Do you go straight to the genitals? Do you feel frustration that you're not 'getting there' fast enough or at all? Brainstorm for yourself, are there things you could do to help you drop into your body and its pleasure before you self-pleasure? Erotic dancing, full body touch, porn, what can you integrate into your pleasure practices so you can really connect with your pleasure and arousal.

The next time you're planning a sexy date with yourself or another, remember the graph, your reactive arousal and look at these things you've brainstormed. Plan a few of these at the start of your connection, to give the person who needs a little more time and attention just that. This is how we all have a better experience, this is how we can ensure a pleasurable experience for all, even with a slower arousal response.

This can be tricky for some people, and the idea of receiving more attention than the other may be surprisingly difficult. We're raised in a culture to believe that sex is some form of an exchange. Well, it's not. You don't give, *just* so you can receive. There should be no agenda in sex. If you need to receive more attention, more touch and more focus in sex, please know you're not a selfish lover. You don't need to 'return the favour'. Sex is a gift and doesn't need to be strictly two-way all the time. Remove the agenda, so you can access your pleasure.

If you drew a comparison graph and the multiple lines on it don't intersect, perhaps one of your lines looks almost horizontal, that's okay. That happens and you're definitely not the only one. Please know that there is hope. You can rehabilitate your arousal and work towards getting those lines to intersect, towards getting your line to move upwards quicker. How? By doing those sensate activities detailed in the 'pleasure is a bicep' section in part 2 or my online course. It's all about neurologically rewiring our pleasure pathways, and those sensate techniques and the strategies in this book can do just that.

If you love the idea of playing with each other, touching and reconnecting, but aren't sure how, remember the list of activities in Part 2. In particular, 'chatty massage', the '2-minute game' or 'active receiving'.

27. UH-OH, WHERE'S MY O? (CHANGES IN ORGASM)

Something not often spoken about is how during and after cancer treatments your orgasms can change, or sometimes even disappear.

I've touched on this in the chemo section; however, this can occur with other treatments. This is common (it happened to me and many others I support), this is normal, you are normal.

How can they change, you ask? Maybe they're less 'intense', maybe they're more intense. Perhaps you need a lot more time and play (yum!) to 'get there', maybe your body shakes and does the things it normally does, but you don't really feel any actual orgasm. What I call a *'ghost-gasm'*, and was very strange to me during chemo when I first experienced this. There is also the possibility that orgasms and climaxes may not be possible for a while. Sex can still be very pleasurable during cancer treatments, but sometimes our medications block that 'peak-climactic' experience.

Thanks to the wonders of neuroscience, we now know that our body can 100% relearn how to have them, or have *different* ones.

Firstly, know that there are multiple potential blockers to

climaxing. If you're on particular antidepressants or other treatments like chemo, maybe had nerve damage from surgeries and other things, climaxing (orgasms) may not be achievable just yet. It's okay, you can still have a *lot* of pleasure. Sex can still be great sex during and after cancer, without the end point, without that 'goal'.

If you would like to relearn how to have orgasms, or better put, if you would like to rewire your pleasure so the body you now have can have climaxes (even if they're a little different) here's something to try.

Regular self-pleasure with a few rules

I'm talking even just 2-5 minutes a day (10 would be better).

1. Remove the goal, remove the pressure

Ban the orgasm. You heard me! You're only allowed to touch and enjoy your body to rewire your brain and associate touch with *'goal-free'* pleasure. This neurologically starts to rewire your brain in the background that intimacy isn't about the pressure of that goal. This creates freedom and can be a major stepping stone to your pleasure and orgasm recovery. Better yet, if you have a partner/s, have a 'no orgasm allowed' touch-fest a few times a week. Even if you currently can't orgasm, removing it verbally anyway allows you to enjoy the touch you're receiving (and it gets better). Remember, removing the goal can help you get to the goal. You can do this with a partner, but if so, put a timer on and you're only allowed to touch while the timer (5-10mins) is on. It's another way to remove that expectation of it having to 'go somewhere'.

2. Don't forget to breathe.

Breath is powerful, as it not only can be used to down or up-regulate our nervous system, but it also aids in circulating blood to our internal tissues. So many of us tense up and hold our breath when we're in pleasure or when we're *trying* to have an intense moment. It's like we're forcing an orgasm to arrive, which is going to get in the way of you having one! It's like trying to force yourself to go to sleep, the effort of forcing it counteracts where you want to go.

Next time you're having pleasure (with yourself or another), relax your muscles and slow down your breath. Remember, this is about pleasure not orgasms, so be curious. Relaxing your body and making sure you're breathing gets blood flow to the deep internal tissues. With blood flow, the tissues get oxygenated and guess what? Our sensitivity increases and so does our pleasure!

If you notice you're tense and/or hold your breath in pleasure, have a few practice runs with yourself. Touch your body, experience pleasure and arousal, but when you notice your muscles tensing up or you're holding your breath, stop, slow down, and only continue when you're relaxed again. Think of it like a pleasure mediation. It can feel strange, but trust me, blood-flow is the key to arousal and pleasure, and we can't circulate blood without breath, and blood can't reach our internal pleasure structures without those muscles being relaxed.

3. Slow it down.

Some of my work includes masturbation coaching with clients, teaching people that there is more than just fast-paced standard movements. When we rush, we get distracted and then that '*should*' brain (the obligation and pressure of getting somewhere) can get in the way. Plus, as just mentioned, going slow allows blood circulation and muscles to relax... again, blood-flow increases our sensation, arousal and our pleasure. Remember how cancer treatments often give us a slower arousal response, so we need more time to really get into it? Orgasms may be achievable; they just need more time and 'warm-up'. If this is you, take a look at the 'toys' section a little later, I have some suggestions for you.

4. Repetition.

To make change neurologically you need time and repetition. Self-pleasure regularly, a few times a week, over months, maybe 5 mins of loving touch every day if you can (but a few times a week if that's more doable for you). Pleasure rewiring is not a quick fix, but from someone who's been-there-done-that after treatments, it can be done!

5. Lastly, TOYS.

Explore with vibration as it offers stimulation to the deeper tissues and in a way we can't offer naturally. It's a great kick-starter for those times when you want to experience pleasure, but aren't sure exactly what your body enjoys. If you're not sure where to start looking (as the range of intimacy toys is endless), refer to the upcoming section titled 'it's toy time'.

Firstly, for people with a vulva, the vagina is not designed to have peak orgasmic experiences, the clitoris is. And although most of our clitoral structure is internal, we do have a portion of it externally/on the outside of our body for easy access. So, you could try stimulating the head of your clitoris (the part of the clitoris you can access on the outside of your body) before and during play as a way to warm-up and kick-start your reactive arousal.

For people with a penis, there are now incredible ranges of vibrators for you, again, more on that in the toys section. Plus, if you're experiencing changes in erection, remember that your delightful soft penis is 100% capable of pleasure and orgasms.

Lastly, please know there is nothing wrong with using toys. Just like we use glasses to read better, we can use toys to pleasure better. And toy shopping with a partner? Best foreplay ever!

A quick note, that there are some countries which legally sell THC and cannabis products and some users tell me that specific strains can influence arousal and their ability to climax. I cannot make recommendations as unfortunately Australia is a little behind and it's not legal here, so I can't access this product. I feel it would be irresponsible of me not to mention this, for those who live in countries and specific states of the US that can access this, and may want to look into it further.

This is very general advice and I know our bodies are much more complicated than a few simple steps, but the information here is truly powerful. Our desire and arousal are so complicated during and after cancer treatments, and also for partners. Be kind to yourselves, this is tough and the changes in your body may well be temporary.

28. OUR POOR VAJOOTZ (VAGINAL PAIN & ATROPHY)

For people with a vulva, genital pain is very common from treatments. To just quickly explain those words if 'vulva' is new to you; the vagina is the internal portion of the genitals. It refers to the internal canal, where things like tampons, toys, fingers and penises can go into. Vulva is the word for the parts of the genitals on the outside; including the labia, vaginal entrance (the vaginal introitus), mons pubis (pubic bone), clitoral hood, shaft and head etc. 'Atrophy' is a medical word for tissues thinning, breaking down or getting weaker. From various treatments (chemo, radio, endocrine, surgeries impacting / removing sexual organs), vulva and vaginal tissues can get 'roughed up' so to speak and cause discomfort and pain.

Words like 'sandpaper', 'burning' or 'glass-shards' are used to describe the pain felt during internal play. And for people like me, pain felt all day every day during even the simplest of things like walking, sitting or simply wearing underwear. Atrophy can interfere with quality of life, with daily function, cause social and romantic isolation, and isn't something to be ignored.

Why you should have caution when you hear 'use it or lose it' regarding vaginal pain

I honestly can't believe how many people are told by healthcare providers "use it or lose it" in regards to painful penetrative sex. Please, *please*, have caution. The "use it or lose it" motto is a statement for people that work in neuroscience. It's used to describe the process of neuroplasticity in regards to neurological rehabilitation, say after brain or spinal cord injury, NOT musculoskeletal issues. It certainly doesn't apply for pain. Being told you should have painful sex to heal the painful sex is like someone telling you that walking on your broken leg will help it heal.

I think what is happening here, is that clinicians know that blood-flow is the number one way to heal tissues, and for the vaginal canal, getting aroused is a way to get blood to that area. Clinicians also understand that the vaginal canal can maintain its elasticity with 'use'. What clinicians seem to be leaving out of this conversation, is the understanding that many of us do not or cannot have vaginal penetration, and that intentionally causing ourselves more pain can be traumatic to ourselves and to our partners. I have supported people who have forced themselves to have painful and unwanted penetrative sexual experiences because they thought it was their only option (quoting this badly-used-motto to me), which has resulted in more damage physically and also psychologically. Speaking from a consent perspective, this is not okay.

There are endless ways to have sex, to get aroused, to get blood flow to your pelvis, and strengthen the internal muscles, all without having to be penetrated/cause you more harm. Remember, pain is your bodies alarm system telling you something is wrong. And, as mentioned in the libido recovery section in part 2, if you're forcing yourself to have painful sex, your brain is going to start to associate sex as something that is bad/negative/painful/a source of anxiety/stressful and you will WANT IT LESS. It's the ultimate libido killer.

Are you still on treatments? If you're still on treatments like endocrine treatments, your atrophy won't completely recover as you're still taking the thing that causes it. But you can totally help improve it a *lot*, which I cover shortly. Also, if you're on endocrine treatments / had internal radiation, the vaginal entrance or canal can shrink a bit, which can be another source of pain. As mentioned in the radiotherapy section, you can use dilators, fingers or toys to maintain canal size and shape, if you wish.

I've been speaking very strongly here, as I see so many people hurting themselves and having negative sexual experiences because they think it's their only option, or that they *should* just force it and grit their teeth through the pain. This isn't helping anyone. So, here are some other options and ways we can lessen vaginal pain and maintain function, without doing more damage.

1. Stop.

As mentioned, please avoid penetrative forms of sex while it hurts, as you'll only make it worse. Remember, pro-tip: Sex should never, ever hurt. As I've said multiple times throughout this book, if we put up with pain and have sex we don't enjoy, we will start associating the act of sex as something that is not enjoyable and, in turn, *want it less.*

2. Chat.

Have someone physically take a look at your vulva and/or vagina for an accurate diagnosis. Someone who knows your treatments, your body, your cancer and what is safe for you. There are other possibilities than just atrophy which can cause vulvovaginal pain, such as vulva eczema, inflamed Bartholin's glands at the vaginal entrance or lichen sclerosis. Seeing a professional for an accurate diagnosis is vital for your recovery and well-being. If you're not satisfied with the recommendations of who you see, you can always seek another medical professional.

3. Moisturise.

Just like we moistures our hands when they're dry and cracked, you'll need to moisturise your vagina. And regularly. There are internal moisturisers of all brands and types, shop around and find what suits you. How often you need to use moisturisers will vary depending on the severity of your atrophy, your type of cancer and your day-to-day functionality, so contacting your doctor, oncologist or gynaecologist is important. Particularly if you have hormone receptive cancer, as some moisturisers can have hormones in them. It's important you talk about what's safe for you.

4. Lube.

The #1 way to know if you likely do have atrophy, is if you feel discomfort and pain during vaginal penetrative sex even when you're using lube.

Why would you still experience pain if you're using lube? If you have vaginal atrophy, lubricants aren't going to help, because the problem isn't friction / needing things to be slippery (which is the sole purpose of lubes), the problem is the health of your internal tissues. Lubes don't fix pain, they prevent it. This is where we need to use internal moisturisers as described above.

I recommend using lubricants even when you aren't experiencing discomfort, because lubes make good things great and reduce friction. But if you're new to buying them, the choices can be overwhelming, so here's some tips.

The human body is an extremely complex organism and is designed to self-heal, so when your internal tissues are dehydrated and damaged, your body sucks up water like a sponge. That's why, when it comes to vaginal atrophy, water-based lubes are *not* the best. If we don't constantly top-up while playing, we're at risk of doing more damage, as we get dry inside quickly (as we've absorbed the water) and that dryness causes rubbing and friction. Plus, some water-based lubes once absorbed leave a residue inside us, and this can actually cause *more* friction than if you weren't using a water-based lubricant at all.

When in doubt, use a silicone-based lube. These are super slick and don't get absorbed into our bodies nearly as fast. Silicone lubricants aren't great to use on silicone toys (as they can break down the toy over time), but that's okay, just pop a latex condom over the toy and you're good to go.

Oil-based lubes are also great like organic coconut oil, as they also last longer. If this language is new to you, I'll cover the types of lubricants that are out there in more detail, shortly in the section titled 'lube is life'.

There is also a wax-based product called 'olive & bee' which is fantastic for anyone experiencing discomfort internally, and can be used as a lubricant *and* an internal moisturiser. The natural wax and olive oil has healing properties and feels great on sore tissues.

Remember, lubes don't help tissues heal, they only prevent doing tissue damage through reducing friction. So, using a moisturiser regularly as well as using lubricants every time you play internally is key.

5. Exercise.

Light exercise such as walking or yoga puts your pelvis in motion and gets blood circulating. It may seem strange, but this can have wonderful benefits for strengthening your pelvic muscles and healing vaginal tissues, as it gets the blood flowing. Try 15-20 minutes per day of brisk walking, but remember anything is better than nothing, so even 5-10 minutes a day will help. If walking isn't your thing, I highly recommend a free online yoga teacher on YouTube. Her channel is called 'Yoga With Adriene' and she has so many fantastic classes and programs, to suit anyone and everyone.

Anything that gets your pelvis moving and the blood flowing is a win, so find what works for you.

6. Pleasure.

Yup, I want you to self-pleasure. Not internally though as it might cause you more pain and increase tissue damage. I mean you or a partner offer pleasure externally. Clitoral stimulation, anal stimulation and other erogenous zones. Arousal gets blood to the deep tissues inside your pelvis and around your genitals, which promotes healing.

Having difficulties getting aroused on your treatments/meds? Use a vibrator on your clitoris and/or anus (more on that later in the 'it's toy-time' section). They work a treat and remember, you can have sex, pleasure and orgasms without having to be penetrated, especially while it hurts.

7. Bathe.

Just as walking is great to get blood-flowing, so is a warm soak in the bath. It relaxes the muscles, the joints and (noticing a theme here?), gets blood to the internal tissues. If you don't have a bath, pop a *warm* (not hot) wheat-pack or *warm*-water bottle between your legs if it feels soothing. It will still get the blood flowing and help heal.

If you're using dilators or other objects to insert into your vaginal canal, getting your body warm and relaxed beforehand can be a lot more comfortable for you.

8. Oil.

Not only can we have internal atrophy, but also external. The vulva tissues on the outside of your body, like your labia and around the vaginal entrance can be sore. Applying some organic coconut oil, or even internal moisturisers on the outside of your genitals after the shower can help replenish the tissues and ease pain. Some people also use organic coconut oil internally as a substitute for an internal moisturiser. Find what's right for you.

9. Underwear.

Breathable, natural and comfortable underwear is important. I switched to 100% natural bamboo underwear as cotton was too painful for me. My vulvovaginal atrophy and pain was so bad I got to the point where I could barely walk, putting my entire life on hold. We're all different, so try a few things out. When I found the right brand for me, I nearly cried from the relief from the pain when I put them on.

And speaking of underwear, with vaginal and vulva atrophy, menstruation for many is a very stressful and painful experience. Sanitary pads, tampons, cups and other insertables can be painful to use and for me, caused of a lot of anxiety. There are however, brands of 'period underwear' with inbuilt absorbent padding and are machine washable. As someone who was skeptical, but gave them a go as tampons were excruciating for me to use, I was pleasantly surprised by how well they work and how comfortable they are. Each country has its own brand, so I won't recommend one specifically, but these are an incredible option to manage menstruation, while avoiding the pain and stress of having to insert anything.

10. Allied Health.

Not only do you have your oncologist, gynaecologist and other specialists on your side, but there are also pelvic floor physiotherapists, osteopaths and occupational therapists who specialise in this. You don't have to do this alone! All countries have their own unique medical and referral systems, but you won't know what's out there and who you can access unless you ask.

A note of caution: There are creams that have numbing agents which can be inserted into the vaginal canal to numb pain, and as incredible as this may sound, I need to ensure you're careful. Just like lubricants, numbing creams don't heal, they simply temporarily numb an area of the body, reducing sensation and pain. So, if you're using a numbing cream say for penetrative sex while you have internal atrophy, you won't feel pain (your body's warning system that it's being hurt), and may do more harm. Some people notice they are in even more pain once the cream wears off, as they have further damaged their tissues. Numbing creams can be used, but it's essential you only use them if advised by your gynaecologist or medical professional who has examined you. You don't want to cause more damage, more pain and in turn, create more stress around sex.

Laser treatments.

In several countries around the world, there are vaginal treatments which use lasers to 'ease' atrophy and its side-effects. I'm yet to read the results of any studies on these treatments, so have no evidence-based perspective on this. I do know some countries have banned this 'treatment' as the lasers were not designed to treat atrophy (hence the lack of evidence that it is safe and appropriate to use), plus the people operating them are not medically trained. Some countries however, have clinics up and running.

I've heard mixed results from people. By mixed I mean it has been wonderful for some and not at all for others. Please don't book a session without chatting with your gynaecologist or oncologist first. They're not cheap and may not be suitable or safe for you. If you've had internal vaginal radiation therapy, internal lasers may not be an option for you, so it's vital for your safety you speak to a gynaecologist.

29. CHANGES IN ERECTION

I've mentioned changes in erection several times in this book, but want to give it more voice and space here. As a sexual organ that is mostly on the outside of the human body and highly visible, changes in penis function can cause a lot of body-shame and anxiety.

I must repeat, that your penis is capable of extreme pleasure without needing to be hard or erect. Orgasms are entirely possible, even if you cannot be erect or ejaculate.

For people who are experiencing changes in function, the resource 'A Touchy Subject' is run by a clinical sexuality and prostate cancer researcher Victoria Cullen. She specializes in penile and sexual health post prostatectomy. In particular her free penis rehab program and the online 'Masterclass' which rehabilitates sensation and function. We collaborated on this project and is getting wonderful sexual outcomes for participants. Victoria offers a broad range of information that is relevant for anyone and everyone with erectile challenges and her work is changing lives for the better.

There are options, sure there's Viagra (which doesn't always work), but there's also pumps and vacuum devices, medications, injections and physical rehabilitation. You don't need to do this alone and your urologist, physiotherapist, oncologist, doctor, Victoria Cullen and I, are all here for you.

30. LUBE IS LIFE (& OTHER SAFETY ITEMS)

I want to march the streets of every major city across the globe, with thousands of chanting companions screaming for the use of lube. Lubricants are one of the most important and most underused sexual aids. Lube is your lovely friend, the friend that is easily and readily available any time you need it. It makes you feel comfortable and safe, and helps you feel good.

I hear some of you say, "But I've never had to use lubricant before. It's never been *needed*," or, "I get my partner/s aroused enough, thanks". Lubricant isn't about mimicking or replacing arousal, it doesn't mean you're doing something wrong; it means you're doing something right. Regardless of your age or your body, lubricant can enhance sexual activity, make it feel better, help it last longer and help make it safer. If sex is toast, lube is the spread. It's a bit like how food tastes good, but add a bit of salt or seasoning and suddenly it's so much better. Some of you might be thinking, "I've always used lube, it's awesome." That's great, keep going!

So, what are they, really? Lubricants are a viscous (slippery) liquid used to reduce friction when two surfaces rub against each other. If you rub your two hands together, fast, right now, you'll hear the sound of the skin rubbing and your hands will get warm (friction does that). Now, put some lube on your hands, maybe some soap and water and rub your hands together again...it's smoother and nicer, isn't it? That's what lubes do, make two surfaces slippery. Lubricants assist with comfort, pleasure and most of all, safety, as it protects your delicate genital and anal tissues. What's more important than our safety?

Safety can mean many things. For anuses, penises or vaginas that are dry or sore, lubricants create extra moisture to relieve friction. Reducing friction and smoothing out surfaces can also *enhance* sensation, it protects barriers like condoms and dams, and most importantly, the moisture helps protect the skin from tearing. Skin tears can be uncomfortable, painful, decrease pleasure and also increase infection risk. Lubricants also reduce the risk of condoms breaking (whether on an object or genitals) as a dry environment can pull/rub on the barrier and strain it, or even tear it. Lubricants contribute to a safer sexual experience, and allow you to relax and enjoy more. If you're using lubricants and you're still feeling discomfort, please speak with your treating team and if you have a vulva & vagina, take a look at the 'our poor vajootz' section.

If it goes in, put it on

The simple rule with lube is this: If anything is going to be inserted anywhere? Make sure it's clean, covered, and use lube.

This includes tampons if you're feeling sore, tight or dry. Lube is nothing to be ashamed of or embarrassed about. Have it on your bedside table loud and proud, it shows you care about your and your lovers' well-being.

In Australia you can buy lubricants at your supermarket, local chemist, corner store and petrol station. If you don't want to buy lubricant in person, not a problem. They are easily purchased online and you can order small tubes/small amounts when you're first finding what you like, to avoid breaking the budget. Plus, online stores have more variety and much better quality than what you generally find in your local shop. Lubricants aren't expensive, so you can try many types to work out which ones you like as it makes a big difference to get a lubricant that suits you.

You can get everything from really basic to super organic to extremely fancy. I's about finding what suits you best, but I'll say this. Lubricants are like aeroplane tickets; you get what you pay for. It can be worth spending a little more for a better experience, especially if you have sensitive skin or atrophy, as the cheaper items may have more chemicals in them and cause a reaction.

What's out there?

There's quite a few different types of lubricants and moisturisers, and it can seem a bit daunting. Don't worry, I've broken it down, so you can find what is good for you.

Water-based:

In Australia you can get these everywhere, and are usable on toys and latex condoms. Water-based lubricants are easily absorbed by our bodies, so it's normal if you need to keep applying. Plus, if you like it very runny, you can also add more water to a water-based lube. Please don't think there is anything wrong if you need to keep adding more during play, it simply means your body is doing what it's designed to do, absorb water. When it comes to water-based lubricants, more is more.

Silicone based:

These lubricants are perfectly safe and are longer lasting, so you don't have to reapply as often as water-based lubes, plus they feel wonderful. The only thing that most silicone lubes are not good for is to use them with silicone toys as it can damage the toy over time. If you're not sure, go to the website of the particular brand you're interested in to see if they specify it is safe to use on a silicone toy or not. Generally found in the FAQ section if their website has one. Sex toys that are made of other materials such as stainless steel, rubber, vinyl or glass are fine with this type of lube. If you want to use a silicone toy with your silicone lube, simply pop a condom over the toy creating a barrier between the two. If choosing is a bit overwhelming, I use Überlube and Sliquid Silver, they're so great.

Hybrid:

This means water-based mixed with silicone, it's a 'hybrid' of the two main types of lubricants out there. These lubes last longer than solely water-based lubes as they're mixed, however they still do get absorbed by the body over time, as there is high water content.

Oil-based:

Oil based lubricants such as organic coconut oil or organic castor oil and more, are used by some and they certainly work as a lubricant skin-to-skin, however there are a few things to mention. Oil-based lubricants can break down some latex materials which means that it's best to avoid oil-based lubricants when barriers (like latex condoms) are being used. You can however, buy condoms that are made out of other materials than latex, which are fine with oil-based products. Also, for those who have a vagina, oil-based lubricants can be thicker and harder for the internal tissues to flush out. I know many people who use organic coconut oil as a lubricant (and is great for massage oil), but have caution as it can cause thrush in some. A way to test this is to put a dab of oil on your inner thigh/outer labia to look for any reactions first.

Wax-based:

I'm referring to a particular product here because wax-based lubes aren't a huge thing (yet), but a pelvic floor physiotherapist created an 'intimate cream' made from beeswax and olive oil called 'olive & bee'. As described in the vaginal atrophy section, it can be used as a lubricant and also as an internal moisturiser. I have a few favourite lubes and moisturisers I like to use and this is in my top three. I use it as both a lubricant and a moisturiser. The beeswax is thick and creates a protective barrier, the olive oil has healing properties and because it's so thick and slick, it's pretty great for people with vulva & vaginal atrophy (hence why I love it so much).

Sterile lubricants:

Generally, water-based, sterile lubes are commonly used in hospitals and clinical settings. It's as the name sounds, sterile. With a lower infection risk, this lube is used by medical professionals and is excellent to use with toys, especially toys/items that will penetrate. Remember me mentioning our very delicate internal tissues? Sterile lubricants can offer that extra layer of safety in case of any tissue damage. They are easily purchased online from medical stores and some online sex stores also. Plus, if you're UTI prone, sterile lubricants can be great as they have such a lower infection risk.

Chemicals:

Avoiding lubricants with high chemical content is recommended. So, don't purchase lubes that are coloured, scented or flavoured. Also, check the ingredient listing on the product label for parabens or other chemically sounding things, as they can irritate the skin. Essentially, if you're reading the ingredients list and you see a word so long you want to buy a vowel in order to be able to read it…..I'd give that word a good old google before buying the product. There are also 100% natural organic options which are easily found online.

Lubricants used for anal-play:

For anal penetration, it's recommended by many in the industry to use thicker, more viscous lubricants (avoid lubricants with glycerin as they can get sticky and create friction). As a very important job of the rectum is to absorb water, silicone-based lubricants can be great for the anus as there is less water in them, so they last longer. There are also water-based lubricants which are thicker and specially designed for anal play, these are also great, but you *must* make sure they specify they are for anal use. Remember, a standard water-based lubricant will be absorbed quickly into your body and you may experience friction if you don't top up regularly.

Whether you're on treatments or not, lubricants are essential as our anuses don't produce moisture on their own, so lubricant makes everything more comfortable. The tissues are quite delicate in there, so if you warm-up your anus (a bit of foreplay doesn't hurt anyone - literally!) and use lubricants, you will avoid causing any damage. As I keep saying, the anus is a highly pleasurable area of the human body and it needs care before being played with.

Vaginal moisturisers:

Are exactly what they sound like. A moisturiser that gets applied inside the vagina, repeatedly over a period of time. Some are only accessible via a script from your oncologist which may contain hormones and others are available at pharmacies on the shelf. Please ask your doctor before purchasing one and speak with the pharmacist when you're there, about the medications you're on. There may be ingredients that will cause a reaction to your internal tissues, the only way to know if something could benefit you, is to consult with your treating team. Some vaginal moisturisers have hormones such as oestrogen in them, so if your cancer is hormone receptive, this may have negative impacts. It may be fine, but better to be sure and safe. You will need to speak to your oncologist to ask if a vaginal moisturiser is appropriate for you to use and they will recommend what is best for you.

There are hormone free moisturisers on the chemist and pharmacy shelves, some need prescriptions from doctors, and others you can order online. If you need a hormone free internal moisturiser, look for anything that contains hyaluronic acid. It's a slick substance we produce naturally in our bodies to keep our synovial joints moving smoothly and it's great for our internal tissues.

There are also moisturisers which can be used externally, for the vulva area. Again, you will need to consult your treating team to see what is recommended as having the right cream is vital to avoid potential harm. This is one of those times where you really must ask.

Using lube with barriers

Lubricants need to be put on after the safer sex barrier is in place. If lube is put on the body part or toy before the barrier, you're creating a slippery surface under the barrier and there is a much greater risk (almost a guarantee) of it coming/sliding off during play.

- If you're using a condom for a penis or toy to be inserted into something, put the condom on first, then the lube on the condom covered penis/toy.

- If you're using an internal condom for a vagina or anus, put the condom inside the person first, then the lube. Also, with internal condoms, the lube can also go on the thing that will penetrate, such as a toy, finger or penis before insertion.

- If you're using a condom for an individual finger, pop the condom over the finger, then put lube over the condom-covered finger.

- Regardless of treatment, if you're going to insert anything, anywhere, put a condom on it and then lube on the condom. This is an extra way to ensure cleanliness and hygiene and also makes cleaning the toy/object/person much easier.

Gloves

Gloves are a wonderful and versatile safer sex item. If you're touching someone's genitals and feel you have dirt under your fingernails or perhaps some cuts and abrasions on your hand/fingers, pop some gloves on. Most importantly, is to mention that gloves don't remove all sensory feedback, as the person wearing gloves, you can still feel plenty.

Gloves also feel excellent on skin, for the person being touched. They're just another way to explore and enjoy new and different sensory experiences. There are several types of gloves, vinyl, latex or Nitrile. Nitrile gloves are easily accessed online and are great for people who have a latex allergy.

31. A QUICK NOTE ON HYGIENE

Self-care regimes during treatments can be exhausting, however it's very important to stay clean to lower infection risk and prevent discomfort. I'm not saying that you need to shower three times a day, but at least once a day is necessary. It's important to keep your body clean and refreshed, but remember, our genitals need particular care as they have such soft and sensitive tissues, and treatments can make our genitals more sensitive and irritated. So, we want them to be clean, but we also don't want to irritate them further with soaps that can wash away all of the protective and amazing natural bacteria we have around and inside our genitals. Too much washing (especially with soaps) can actually cause more irritation, so here's some tips.

- Wipe after going to the toilet
  - Those with a vulva, wipe front to back
  - Those with a penis, gently pat dry
- Wash your genitals with warm (not hot) water. Avoid using things like a flannel or sponge, as they can scratch and irritate the skin.
- As with lubricants, also avoid perfumed soaps or soaps that have chemicals. Warm water is usually sufficient, but

if you want to use soap, make sure it's pH balanced and specifies on the label that it's for 'intimate areas'. This applies for all genital configurations. These soaps are available on the shelf in Australian chemists and supermarkets (and online anywhere in the world).

- The vagina has a self-cleaning system, which is why we so often have discharge in our underwear. If you notice a change in smell, please don't use soaps internally, continue to wash externally with warm water and let your vagina clean itself out as it's designed to do. If things don't seem quite right, chat with your doctor.

- Similarly, don't use soap directly on the head of a penis or under a foreskin. Retract the foreskin, wash with warm (not hot) water and then replace the foreskin.

- When you're drying yourself after a shower or bath, gently pat your genitals dry with your clean towel. You want to avoid rubbing and scraping type motions.

- Avoid perfumes and deodorants in those areas and looser fitting clothing can help the skin breathe if you're feeling sensitive.

- If you use pantyliners, change them regularly and only use when needed. They're not for everyday use as they trap in warmth and moisture. Period underwear breathe and are great if you change them each morning and night.

Haemorrhoids and anal fissures

Warning, Tess over-share coming! My cancer treatment side-effects and impacts were endless. From my first type of chemotherapy, the oh-so appropriately nicknamed 'red devil' I experienced severe constipation, causing haemorrhoids and anal fissures. Then, when I switched to the weekly "not-so-shit" chemo as my oncologist called it, I had chronic diarrhoea - causing more haemorrhoids. And just when I thought it couldn't get any worse, with that new chemo I also experienced constant sneezing fits. Let's think about that for a second. Diarrhoea and sneezing…it was *almost* comical. Anal health and care are a part of my daily routine, not only so I can go to the toilet without crying, but so I can also access pleasure.

There are many topical creams available to treat hemorrhoids, ask your doctor/GP, pharmacist or oncologist what they recommend. A warm, Epsom salt bath can soothe haemorrhoid pain and also relax the sphincters and surrounding muscles. Generally, avoid any anal play until your pain eases and then, please use lubricants. Lubricants are an anuses best friend. If you're using condoms, you have two choices: the regular external condom, AKA the 'male condom' that rolls onto toys and penises, and the internal condom AKA the 'female condom' that can fit inside the anus (and vagina's). Not many folks have heard of the internal condom, but they're available from some chemists, online sex stores and from STI clinics. They're also useful for smaller penises or ones that aren't as hard, and they also offer a different sensation to a standard condom. No matter what you're using, remember that nothing should be inserted anally (even a fingertip) without lubricant.

There are also some anal exercises you can do, to strengthen the sphincters and increase blood flow to the area, which can have positive impacts (I noticed less pain within a day doing this). This may seem strange, but the anal sphincters are connected to our pelvic floor muscles and if they are healthy, able to relax and contract? Not only may pain improve, but also blood flow can increase, which influences healing, arousal and pleasure.

A few exercises are:

1. As you breathe in, clench your anus shut. As you breathe out, relax it (or the opposite way if that feels more right for you). The release is just as (if not more) important than the clench. The release is the motion that allows blood flow to access the tissues.

2. As you breathe in, clench your anal sphincter about half-way, pause, then clench all the way to as hard as you can. Like a two-step clench on the inhale. And then relax on your exhale.

3. Clenching and release your anal sphincter with breath, but much faster.

Do these a few hundred times a day (I'm quite serious) and you may experience improvements such as less pain or going to the toilet easier. To make sure you remember to do it, you could remind yourself to do these exercises when you do a certain daily activity, such as every time you open the fridge, do twenty. Or do 30 when you sit down for a coffee, are stopped at a traffic light or when you go to bed.

If you have had any type of bowel, rectal or pelvic surgery, please have a discussion with your surgeon / oncologist / doctor / pelvic floor physiotherapist before you start doing any exercises. Pelvic floor physiotherapists are incredible for regaining strength in this area.

If you experience pain when doing any pelvic floor/anal strengthening exercises, stop doing them immediately and speak with your treating team. And of course, if you're in pain and topical ointments are not helping, see a doctor.

Things to buy/consider

There are many, many online stores where you can buy products such as condoms, gloves, lubricants, accessories, toys and countless other items. Don't fear ordering something for delivery and it showing up in the post with a massive picture of someone's genitals on it screaming 'SEXY STUFF IN HERE!' It's not in the interests of the online intimacy store to embarrass or 'out' a customer. In Australia, packages are delivered in non-descript boxes that look like any other package to the postal worker and credit card statements have very common, nondescript names. And while I'm at it, there are many walk-in sex stores that are clean, well-lit and have super friendly staff to answer questions. It's like going into an Apple store, but with better toys. Going into a sex store can be handy if you'd like a chat with the staff to see what might suit you best. Of course, during treatments like chemotherapy and radiotherapy, getting to your appointments is draining enough, so online shopping can still have a lot of information about each toy, and save you the effort of physically having to move.

32. SEXUAL POSITIONS, TECHNIQUES & TOOLS

If you haven't yet realised, I love being an OT. We're 'out of the box' thinkers and are also extremely practical, which is why my ADHD brain loves and suits the profession so much. We look at how brains function and how body's function. We see daily activities as not just an activity, but a series of tasks and actions and sequences that make up that activity, which are influenced not only by how our body and brain are working at the time, but also the surrounding environments, contexts, who you are as a person and your values. When we look at functional activities and the many tasks that contribute to that activity being completed (like sex), we break things down and reshape those tasks in a way that suits our clients' needs. Enabling them to best do that activity around their limitations and functionality. We don't care if the way you do something doesn't look the same as the way other people do that thing, what we care about is the fact that you're able to do it! Alright, enough gushing. This section is where I really wear my OT hat and discuss positioning.

Sex as a functional activity is extremely adaptable, with so many possible positions we can put our bodies in and so many adaptations to suit our needs. Here, I offer some suggestions and ways to alter the positions of your body to get around some of the trickier side-effects of treatments.

Explore, experiment, but make sure you do it from a place of communication and curiosity. You all want to be comfortable and, most importantly, safe, so have a chat beforehand with your lover. Treat it like a brainstorm, note what parts of your body are sore or might need support and figure out how to work around them comfortably and safely. It mightn't seem 'sexy' at first, but these conversations will get easier, and it will make things *much* better. And remember, if it's good, you'll want it more.

DISCLAIMER: These positions are to be used as a guide, not direct clinical recommendations. Please consult your treating team regarding precautions and care relative to your body, and feel into what is right for you, before trying something new. Remember, ask your medical team about any physical restrictions or limitations you may have during and after treatments relative to your symptoms and situation, especially after surgeries. We're all different and only your healthcare team can give you advice specific to you.

And finally, let your pain be your guide, and stop as soon as you feel any discomfort.

Positions for fatigue, lack of energy & oxygen users

The idea of being intimate with someone when your mind and body is fatigued can seem bewildering. Finding a position that doesn't need too much energy is very important. If you're using oxygen, not using too much energy is a way to avoid losing your breath. Sex can be soft, slow, gentle and warm (and still be hot). You don't have to have a full body work-out to have a beautiful connection. Let someone else do the work.

Remember that fatigue diary I recommended you keep? This is when it comes in handy, to find those times during the day/week/treatment cycles where you have more energy. We want to use it for pleasure, not for chores! Essentially, you'd want to position the person using oxygen or who is fatigued, in a position that doesn't involve much muscle engagement or movement. Lying on your back, lying on the side or sitting up with your back propped up on a couch or in bed against the wall can involve very little movement and still be intimate.

Being on all fours and having someone behind you can also be done with little energy spent by the person 'receiving'. Stack some pillows on top of each other and pop them under the person's chest so they are still on their knees, but resting on the pillows, rather than holding themselves up. You could even try leaning on or bending over some furniture, while someone can access your yummy behind. These positions are very handy if the other person with you is able to do most of the energetic work, but remember, sex doesn't have to be an Olympic sport to be enjoyable. If both people have low energy, the side-lying position can be great, like a snuggly spoon position.

A wonderful oral sex position, if both people need to use as little energy as possible, or are wheelchair users is with both lying down. How it works is someone lies on the bed on their side, with knees together and bent towards the chest exposing their genitals, like a fetal or right-angle position. The other person, can then lie down on their side and their face can easily access the other persons genitals, both people are lying down and using a lot less energy than other oral sex positions. You can also try a '69' position, but lying on your sides. Imagine a 'lazy-69'.

Plus, hot OT tip here. The more supported and still you are, the less energy you use, so propping yourself up with cushions / leaning against things uses less energy than holding yourself up, and gives you more energy for the fun-stuff.

Positions for nausea

Having your head above your heart can be relieving, or at least, not make nausea worse. Sexual positions that involve someone sitting up or leaning against something and standing are recommended. Sitting on the couch raised on cushions, standing and bracing yourself while you lean over on a kitchen bench/chest of drawers for stability. For oral sex, standing/leaning back into the corner of a room while the other person kneels on the floor in front of you can work well, as the two corners act as a brace each side of you. This allows you to worry less about keeping still, and enjoy what is happening more. Try, timing things around when your anti nausea meds are working their best or even having a snack on some bland foods before getting intimate, to help settle your stomach.

Positions for stomas and catheters

Attention! Sex is still possible if you have a stoma bag/catheter.

For stomas, a helpful tip is to empty the bag before you start and there are smaller pouches which can be worn for 'intimate moments'. Positioning yourself or your lover to reduce the risk of pressure on the bag is helpful. The standard missionary position can be fine, if the person on top has the upper body strength to hold themselves up. Other positions, such as playing with someone from behind or standing up while someone is lying on the edge of the bed or chair can work well to avoid bumping and putting pressure on the bag. The spooning position is also wonderful for people with stoma bags and catheters, as the person in the front has more space in front of them. There are many, well-designed intimate-wear options for all genders, for those who have stoma bags and are self-conscious about it showing.

For catheters, before any sexual activity, emptying the urine collection device and securing it out of the way is recommended. For those with a penis, you can fold the catheter tube down the penis shaft and cover your penis and tube together with a condom, which holds them together in place and penetration is still very achievable. Just make sure you have enough spare tube at the top for your erection to grow/penis to expand with blood-flow and afterwards, wash and secure it back in place. For those with a vulva, taping the catheter tube out of the way on the abdomen / thigh keeps it out of the way. Having a wash afterwards is recommended (to avoid UTIs) and securing it back in place.

Positions for self-consciousness

As discussed previously our bodies change and so is the way we see ourselves, which can interfere with our sex. Talking about it, is the number one approach with this to explain how you're feeling. I spoke with a husband and wife recently and she told me she had refused to get naked in front of her husband for the entire time since cancer diagnosis from self-consciousness (a period of years). She regrets it now as they have spoken about it since, and all he wanted was to hold his partner and love her. Even just naming the elephant in the room can be such a relief, and then thinking about other options can come.

Wearing clothes / lingerie during sex if you're not wanting to be completely naked is a simple method to ease self-consciousness. There's no shame in wearing a t-shirt during sex, nor a skirt / sarong wrapped around the waist. If you're not ready to look into your lovers' eyes during sex? Try the side-lying position which is like a 'spoon', or someone being taken from behind, or even sitting on your partners lap/being sat on, with the person on top facing away. You could also, under the covers, self-pleasure yourselves, but together, or offer pleasurable touch to each other while under the covers and the lights low. This is still sex.

It's important to note, bodies are complicated and what might work one day, might not the next. It's okay, it's normal, but you need to communicate how you're doing during and after sex. Telling your lover that you're needing to change position because the sheet is rubbing on your chemo rash, or that your muscles are starting to get tired, that you need to slow down due to a bit nausea, or perhaps a drain tube is getting bumped, is important for both of your enjoyment. Comments like this, is you being great at sex. Make the adjustments you need, see if everyone is doing okay, keep going if you're all comfortable and check in after.

If you want to stop, then stop. Remember, don't force it, don't put up with pain, self-pleasure is always there for a partner if someone wants to continue. Hey, if you stop sex as it's a bit too difficult or is no longer pleasurable and your lover wants to continue pleasure through touching themselves? Offer them a hand!

Key positional tricks.

- The more still and supported you are, the less energy you use.

- Having your chest exposed (not against something or someone) can make it easier to breathe.

- Sitting up, and being still is great for people using oxygen and for nausea.

- Having your chest open and staying upright can be more comfortable if you're experiencing acid reflux.

- A pillow under your hips raises the pelvis, allowing easier access to the genitals / anus and also supports the lower back.

- A pillow between the thighs can be wonderful for hip & knee joint pain.

- A pillow/cushion between the knees separates the thighs and prevents them rubbing together if you have sensitive skin there or a catheter taped to your inner thigh.

- If you're standing up and playing with someone lying on a bed / chair, whether they're on their front or back, you can put some pillows underneath them to raise their pelvis to match the height of yours. This avoids you needing to bend / squat down. This is a great tip if you're playing with / penetrating an anus.

- Empty your stoma bag / urine collection device before sex and while you're getting used to it. Try positions that leave space around that area such as standing, sitting, lying on your side, being behind someone, or on top of someone.

- If you have a catheter, stoma or drain-tube, communication is key. Chat, brainstorm, explore, you'll be fine!

- If you have tubes or surgery sites, don't lie on them, use cushions to protect them and lie on your other side (your 'unaffected' side) to avoid pushing / putting weight on them.

- Standing or sitting in a corner has more stability than leaning against a flat wall.

- If you're having sex and are using a manual wheelchair? Double check the breaks are on!

- With any wheelchair play, pop the armrests up / take them off if able, it frees up a *lot* of space.

- If you're uncomfortable deep inside? Use an 'Ohnut' to reduce the depth of penetration.

- If you find a good position, but it's hard to hold yourself in it? Prop yourself up with cushions or pillows.

- Sore joints? Have a bath beforehand or a warm shower and get straight into a warm cosy bed.

- Concerns about continence if you get excited? Having sex in the shower rinses away any urine or faeces that might come out. Avoid using plastic bed sheets as they don't absorb anything and can create more mess. You can pop a towel down on the bed, plus there are great absorbent mats designed for children that wet the bed. I have one, it's machine washable and it's the best.

- Use lubricants, always and forever.

- Get comfy, put cushions under any knees or bums if you're on the ground.

- Lastly, and most importantly, communicate before, during and after about how you're doing.

How to say it out loud.

- "Can we please pause for a second? I just need to re-adjust these cushions, thanks!"

- "I'd love to keep going, but we may need to brainstorm a new position as I'm a bit nauseous / tired / out of breath / sore…"

- "I'm really loving this, could we slow down a bit? I'm

losing my breath."

- "This is so great, but I'm having a hot flush, can we sit up so I'm not in so much contact with the bed?"

- "I'm really enjoying this; I just need to top up the lube."

- "It's wonderful to connect with you, but I'm starting to feel a little dry, can you pass the lube please?"

- "Pause, lube top-up!"

- "I'm feeling some discomfort / changes in my erection, how do you feel about some pleasuring with my hands?"

- "I may need to stop; would you like to continue with self-pleasure? Would you like me to touch your body while you pleasure yourself?"

- "Can we please pause? I'm feeling a bit odd and need a moment, thank you."

- "I don't want to keep going as we are, but really want to continue being intimate with you. Is there some form of different touch or pleasure you might enjoy that I can offer you?"

- "How could you/we enjoy this more?"

- "Is there a speed or pressure of touch that you might enjoy more?"

- "How could this be even better for both of us?"

- "I just wanted to check in, are you comfortable?"

- "Please let me know if you need to change positions at

any time."

- "Please call out for more lube if/when you need, it's within arm's reach."

- "I'm loving connecting with you, I just want to make sure you're comfortable?"

- "I know I'm not moving much, but I'm really enjoying this and I'd like to keep going."

Communicating after intimacy (aftercare).

- Thank you so much, that was wonderful. Is there anything you need or would like in this moment?

- Can we please cuddle for a while? I'd like to stay connected with you for a bit longer.

- I'd love to know what you enjoyed about that experience, and I'll share the same.

- I'd love to know if there was anything you might like to do differently next time, or explore more, and I'll share the same.

- Can we lie here together while I catch my breath?

- This has brought up a few emotions, I'm okay, but chatting for a short while would be lovely.

33. IT'S TOY TIME!

In this section, I'm going to be discussing a few toys out there. I'll never be able to cover it all as it's endless. So, I'm only going to be chatting about a few *types* of toys that I often recommend to clients, who are experiencing changes in their arousal and pleasure.

Firstly, and most importantly. Toys don't mean something is wrong, toys mean something is right! Think of it, the word 'toy' is perfect. It's about fun, it's about play. Approaching sex with playfulness, exploration and curiosity is how to ensure you have a good time on so many levels.

I'm going to start with vibration, as it's a wonderful tool to use for people that have mismatched desire and delayed arousal, and can be a very useful (and fun) way to get someone into their pleasure quicker.

Vibration

Toys that vibrate have a few main purposes which are to offer heightened stimulation and to access deeper tissues. There are countless types of vibration toys and I'll cover a few, but remember this. Vibration is a wonderful method to offer a type of stimulation to parts of our body that we can no longer stimulate ourselves and also offers stimulation in a way we cannot do naturally or anymore. Plus, vibration is felt *deeper* in the body, so it can be more arousing because it reaches more tissues internally. If we're experiencing numbness or changes in sensation and pleasure, exploring with vibration can be a way to stimulate our arousal, when things aren't working the same as they used to.

There are vibrators for penises, vaginas, anuses, the clitoris and there are so many to choose from.

They can be used at the beginning of play, to kind of kick-start pleasure and arousal. They can be used during play, to maintain arousal or increase pleasure. They can be used at the end of play, if perhaps someone wants to heighten their pleasure in the hopes of reaching climax with another partner, or to 'finish-off'.

Or all of the above.

They're also great for vaginal atrophy, that dry sandpaper feeling internally during penetrative sex, as vibrations applied externally on your body (say on the head of your clitoris) stimulates blood flow to the area. Vibration can also be great for people that have changes in genital sensation and may be experiencing 'numbness' and can be a great way to 'wake up' the sensory receptors.

There is no right or wrong way to use them, as long as you're exploring and going slowly the first few times you play with them. When our bodies change, so does our sensitivity, so we can 'overload' ourselves if we go too fast too soon.

I'm going to now introduce you to a very popular vibration toy called the 'doxy wand'.

Doxy massager wand:

The original model was a 'Hitachi wand', which is almost identical to the 'doxy wand', known to be one the most intense vibration toys that exist and were originally designed for deep tissue massage. There are many models available including less expensive ones with a slightly less powerful motor (I think if you type in Amazon or eBay 'body massager' you'll find a bunch). These toys are not designed for internal use, but the vibration is so strong you feel it throughout your whole body regardless.

This toy is wonderful when being held against a vulva, clitoris, anus and that magical perineal space between the scrotum and anus or between the vagina and anus. You *must* start slowly, at the lowest setting. If you start at a higher setting you may get overwhelmed. This is also wonderful for massage and if you're getting intimate with a partner and offering sensual touch, pop this out and use it for relaxation. It's amazing on the lower back and shoulders and helps me get through migraines when I use it on my neck.

Tip #1; When you're using it, pop a condom over the head and a few drops of lube. That way when you're done you can simply pull the condom off and give it a wash in soapy warm water and it's perfectly clean. Plus, with the lube it just makes things smoother and more enjoyable (we always want to prevent friction).

Tip #2; You can use this toy through your hand by placing it on the back of your hand while you're touching someone. This is the toy that can magically turn your hand or fingers into a vibrating hand! And yes, it most definitely does feel good (a friend of a friend told me).

Clitoral vibrators:

Another amazing vibratory toy which also uses air-pulses is a clitoral vibrator.

These toys vibrate and gently suck and pulse air. Anyone using this *must* start at the lowest setting and go slowly, as you want to find what's right for your body. This can be used on a clitoris, the head of a penis (soft or hard) or the nipples. Again, use a few drops of lubricant on the area you're pleasuring.

You can find these toys (there's a few brands) online by searching the word 'clitoris' or 'clitoral vibrator' and they'll come up.

These toys are great for mismatched libido and for anyone

and everyone with delayed/reactive arousal. They feel absolutely **sensational** and are small enough to be used during play. You could use this toy holding it onto your clitoris if you're being taken from behind, or the reverse cow position also. This is a really handy toy to have when someone may need a little more time and pleasure to get aroused. Just be curious, go slow and get to know it. I'm yet to recommend this toy to someone and have them report back to me as anything but happy.

Vibrators for penises:
They do exist in varied forms. I will, however, recommend ones that cup around, or somewhat surround the penis. This way, it can be used for both soft or hard penises and offers better stimulation. Remember, vibration is an internal stimulator and can offer people with soft penises incredible pleasure. It's all about exploring. The 'mantra' and the hot-octopuss 'guybrator' are two which seem to make many people happy.

Anal toys

There are so many varieties of anal toys and I could speak on the topic of anal pleasure forever (and do when I'm running anal-pleasure workshops), so I'm going to keep this super basic.

Most people have had a bad anal experience in sex, for various reasons and most people I coach, feel that because they didn't enjoy it then, means they don't enjoy it at all. I've been continually saying throughout this book that the anus is capable of extreme pleasure, that it needs to be relaxed to be ready (like the rest of our body) for play and penetration. Start with gentle massage, hold some vibration on the outside of the sphincter (like using the doxy wand resting against your finger, so your vibrating fingertip is stimulating the anal entrance), give your body and mind time to relax.

Always start with the smallest toys. Buy the smallest butt-plug and only put the tip in, get used to the sensations. In the shower when you're washing, give the outside of your anus a few moments of soft curious touch.

Vibrating butt-plugs are *amazing* and are great for getting blood to that area. Always start small, start slow, start with curiosity. Bigger is not better, what's good for you is what's right for you.

The blindfold

Yes, this is a sex toy, as well as an object of daily function. This simple and easily found item is a real game changer.

The blindfold can really help quiet that brain-chatter by removing visible distractions and is great to help calm our mind when we're anxious or self-conscious. Plus, when we remove one of our senses, all of the others get heightened. Touch just gets better with a blindfold on. Through decreasing distraction and increasing your sensitivity, this can be a great way to find those erogenous and pleasure zones you never thought existed for greater pleasure. I highly recommend.

So, we've covered some basics in what is an endless topic. Remember, toys are exactly that, toys. They are fun! But also have a lot of benefits post cancer diagnosis as mentioned previously.

I haven't attached links to specific stores online, so you don't think I'm recommending things to simply make a buck. I'm recommending what I know to be beneficial.

If you're not sure where to start, google 'online sex toy store (and your city/country name)'. You will find some.

Check posting to your country, read the reviews online and if they have it available, watch any short videos on how to use the toy.

The international online toy store 'Lovehoney' has lots of 1–2-minute videos on their toys, if you're interested to shop and learn. This can seem a little daunting, but just like everything else in sexuality, approach it with curiosity and exploration, you'll be fine.

34. WHAT HAVE WE COVERED?

- A broader view of treatments and their impacts.

- More communication, but very sex specific.

- How to address sexual shame and communicate that with others.

- Saying 'sex' out loud doesn't make the world explode.

- Some sex-myth busting so you can have more freedom to play and explore.

- Delayed arousal responses and how we can work with them for mutual enjoyment.

- Navigating changes in orgasms.

- Vaginal atrophy, what it is and what we can do.

- The supports that are out there for changes in erection and how it isn't the end of your sex.

- Some information on lubricants and hygiene, so things can be even better.

- Ways to position yourself in sex, for various common side-effects and some general positioning tips to let you get creative and adaptive on your own.

- Some of the toys/intimacy aids that are out there and how they can be useful for our intimacy recovery.

WHERE TO FROM HERE?

Because there is limited work out there on sexuality and cancer and well, actual realistic and accessible sexuality education in general, resources can be hard to find. So, here are some, of varied mediums depending on what suits you best.

An online program for couples

'Connection & Cancer: Reclaim your intimacy & desire'.

www.connectionandcancer.com/course4couples

If the information in this book made sense, but you would like support through the exact steps of *how* to neurologically recover your pleasure, intimacy and libido, then this is for you. It's online, so is done in the privacy of your own home, filled with information and activities, with me guiding you every step of the way. The people who I've worked with in this program are having life-changing results. It's an absolute honour to guide people to recover what they felt was lost forever.

You can find me at:

- **'ConnectAble Therapies'** www.connectabletherapies.com. For consultations and further resources on sex, intimacy & cancer.

- **Facebook** business page *'ConnectAble Therapies'*, where I regularly share information and answer questions.

- **Facebook global support group**: *'Intimacy and Cancer'*. This group is for any cancer, any gender and is a very supportive space.
- **YouTube Channel** on sex, intimacy & cancer: *'Intimacy and Cancer'*. If you prefer video formats over reading (as cancer-brain & reading don't go well together), this YouTube Channel is filled with short videos discussing all things on sex, intimacy and cancer.

'A Touchy Subject' www.atouchysubject.com

For people with prostate cancer or experiencing changes in erection. Victoria Cullen is *the* person to go to, about sexuality and intimacy post a prostate cancer diagnosis. She also has a YouTube channel and through her website access to free resources and rehabilitation programs.

'The Art of The Hook Up' www.artofthehookup.com

This site from dating expert and communication extraordinaire is by Georgie Wolf. Not cancer specific, but incredibly on-point and with relative information for anyone struggling with the dating scene. She has podcasts, blogs, eBooks and more. She's also a workshop facilitator and a bit of a superstar here in Australia!

'Curious Creatures' www.curiouscreatures.biz

For online workshops and much more education on self-development and sexuality. They provide articles, podcasts and streamable workshops which are all very practical and very accessible. I have the privilege to work for this company, their work is changing lives.

Pelvic and sexual health osteopath

For those who live in Melbourne, Australia, we have one of the top pelvic health osteopaths you'll ever find. Dr Andrew Carr from *'Supporting Presence Osteopathy'* is referred to as *'the body whisperer'* in clinical and sexual health circles. He works with the entire body, however has expertise and clinical focus on pelvic and sexual health. In particular, people experiencing pelvic pain including after treatments, vaginismus, atrophy and is trauma informed.

If you're not located in Melbourne, there are pelvic floor osteopaths, physiotherapists and OTs all over the world. Simply search online "Pelvic floor osteopath/physio/OT (insert the name of your city/town here)". You'll find someone near you.

Support groups in your area

If you search in google "Cancer Support (insert city/town where you live here)", there should be a list of businesses and companies that have programs near you. Some online or in person. They mightn't be sexuality specific, but there is always opportunity for discussions and learning.

ABOUT THE AUTHOR

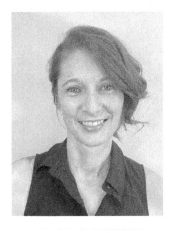 Tess Devèze is an occupational therapist (OT) having completed their bachelor degree in Melbourne Australia. Alongside being an OT, Tess is also a sexuality educator & workshop facilitator, and has facilitated thousands of people in the topics of communication, consent, sexuality, pleasure and relationship dynamics for nearing a decade. They have also completed trainings via the Institute of Somatic Sexology.

Tess is the founder of ConnectAble Therapies, a private community OT practice focussing solely on sexuality for people living with disability, chronic illness and cancer. They educate and advocate for sexual rights for these and LGBTQIA+ communities, which they proudly belong to.

Tess was diagnosed with stage 3 breast cancer at the age of 36 and is still undergoing treatments.

Find them at www.connectabletherapies.com

DID YOU ENJOY THE BOOK?

As an independent author and clinician, my work survives through your support. There are so many people affected by cancer, suffering in silence. With each review or word-of-mouth recommendation you make, we can reach the many out there who are struggling and need support.

Please leave a review by visiting www.amazon.com.au

Got feedback? I'd love to hear from you. You can reach me via email at tess@connectionandcancer.com.

Tess Devèze

Made in the USA
Las Vegas, NV
18 May 2022